ALL ACROSS AMERICA WOMEN ARE RAVING ABOUT ROSEMARYGREEN'S
DIARY OF A FAT HOUSEWIFE . . .

"Your book touched me deeply. Your honesty and candor, and your insight into obesity, will change the lives of many people for the better. You have made a difference in this world."
—Laurie in California

"Your book and your story have given me an inspiration that I have never had before. I am armed and ready to handle my food addictions [because] I identified with so many of the things you wrote about. I want to thank you, Rosemary, for writing this book."

—Lisa in Washington

"I can't thank you enough! Fat or thin, you are a wonderful person. There really is such a thing as addiction to food. Since I finally faced this, I've been able to handle it much better. The new you has made a believer out of me."
—Terri in Oregon

"You have rendered a great service to all of humankind! The inspirational message contained within is enough to coach me through another exercise workout, to sa___ to a food that drives me to binge, and to refu___ ___ ___ ___-ings. I can't thank you enough."

"You are an inspiratio___ ___ ___ ___ heart on the line to h___

"I thank God for your su___ ___ ___ ___urage, and for your being our voice, the ___ ___ obese women in pain. You have opened a door for me and I know I can be free from this obesity."
—Renee in Ohio

more . . .

"As I read your book, you sounded so much like me, the same feelings and fears. I am going to reread it over and over again because I can relate to every page. Thank you for such a wonderful book."

—Ella in Massachusetts

"Thank you! I laughed and cried as I read your diary—so much of it could have been me. You definitely made me feel less alone in the pain. I know you'll be an inspiration to many obese people, as you are to me."

—Roseann in Pennsylvania

"I am a new person because of your book. I'm going to read it and reread it! Your book is the only thing that has truly woken me up."

—Lori in Florida

"Truly inspirational. This should be required reading for everyone involved in an overweight person's life."

—Dayna in Massachusetts

"I cried, laughed, and sympathized with you. Thank you for the inspiration. I've told my friends, patients, and family about your book. They all learned from it."

—Giovanna in Florida

Copies of these testimonials are on file and may be examined at Warner Books, 1271 Avenue of the Americas, New York, NY 10020

DIARY

of a *Fat*

HOUSEWIFE

ROSEMARY GREEN

WARNER BOOKS

A Time Warner Company

The information in this book reflects the author's experiences and is not intended to replace medical advice. Any questions regarding your individual health, general or specific, should be addressed to your physician.

Before beginning any exercise program or nutritional regimen, consult your physician to be sure it is appropriate for you.

WARNER BOOKS EDITION

Copyright © 1995 by Rosemary Green
All rights reserved.

Cover design by Rachel McClain

Warner Books, Inc
1271 Avenue of the Americas
New York, NY 10020

 A Time Warner Company

Printed in the United States of America

Originally published in hardcover by Warner Books.

First Paperback Printing: March, 1996

10 9 8 7 6 5 4 3 2 1

In the beginning, I dreamed of being
the devoted mother by dedicating this book
to my children.
They have suffered much with me.
Then I thought, I will be the great
romantic by dedicating it
to my husband,
whose remarkable patience and
love have literally kept me alive at times.
But finally, I decided to give up devotion
and romance and dedicate the book
to me!
Me, whose very soul is entwined
round every page.

Acknowledgments

Charles Brower stated it perfectly: "Few people are successful unless a lot of other people want them to be." Throughout the production of my diary, I have been blessed to be surrounded by supportive people. It is impossible to name everyone, but special thanks go to:

Colleen Howard, RN, Susan Davis, Constantine Kanelis, and Dr. David Franck for reading the initial draft of my diary and offering their candid feedback.

Kerri Fackrell, who did the artwork for the query package that attracted Warner Books as my publisher.

Natalie Brown, who taught me much about word processing and entered on computer the first 100 pages of my handwritten manuscript.

Clint Brown and C. Wade Brown, Ph.D., who read and edited my diary and offered excellent advice and much needed encouragement.

Deanna DeLong, who believed in me and my diary from the very first moment I discussed it with her. She was a major help in editing the manuscript and preparing the query package.

Jeanmarie LeMense, my very own "fairy godmother" at

Warner Books, who first saw something special in my diary.

Mark Lind, my brother, whose premature death breathed new life into my resolve to conquer my own out-of-control behavior.

Colleen Kapklein, my editor at Warner Books, who masterfully whittled down my diary to an acceptable number of pages.

Debra Womack, my sister and friend. Debra read the rough manuscript, told me which parts I must never think of publishing, and through the years provided me with lots of funny experiences to write about.

Barbara Myers, my sister, my friend. She has cheered me on as no one else, and she has "put her money where her mouth is" many times. I love her.

Stephen Lind, my brother, who inspired me to finally put my diary in print, challenged me to quit eating chocolate, gave me a video camera to record my weight loss, and showed excitement over every little success I achieved.

Elita Lind, my mother, who from my childhood instilled in me a love for reading . . . and writing.

Roy Lind, my father, who taught me how to work.

Conard and Ilah Green, my in-laws, who have shown me more love than I could have ever imagined—regardless of my weight. One day I told them that I needed a computer in order to realize the dream of publishing my diary—but that I was flat broke! Within twenty-four hours, a state-of-the-art computer and printer were delivered to my home. Their quiet love and belief in me has kept me from quitting . . . many times!

Jeremy, Jennifer, Matthew, Tiffany, and Tyler, my children. Only they know the full extent of what my obesity has cost them. Only they know the countless hours they have contributed to the publication of this diary. Never once have I heard a complaint from any of them. My most precious children, thank you for your many sacrifices!

Allen, my husband. His loyalty to me and this book has been phenomenal. He has been my photographer, my literary agent, and chief editor. His clever wit and creativity were magnified tenfold as we experienced the magic of synergy together. He spurred me on when I had no more energy. He loved me when I was unlovable. He (most of the time) remained calm when I was frantic or frustrated or furious. I love him like the words to *our song*, "More than the greatest love the world has known. . . ."

The Fattest Day

by
Rosemary Green

Okay, world, this is it. This is the day.
Nothin' or no one's gonna get in my way.
No more excuses; pullin' out every stop!
I'm ready to soar now, straight to the top.
So trouble and worry, don't even try it . . .
'Cuz nothin's gonna make me get off of my diet!
No rotten husband, no stinky kid punk,
Not even my bedroom that's crammed full of junk.
No dirty diaper, no sticky spilled mess,
Or a silly old notice from the IRS.
Not a new outbreak of the chicken pox
Or a husband needing a pair of clean socks.
Not a filthy oven or a broken jar,
Lipstick on the wall or a smashed-up car.
Not a stained best dress or a burned-up dinner . . .
I mean, *nothin's* gonna keep me from gettin' thinner!

Like everyone else, I've had my full share
Of life's little problems—every worry and care.

And when things are the pits, I respond like a dunce:
"Oh, I must have a candy bar—*at once*!"
The kids are all screaming? Quick! Jump in the car
And go calm yourself down with a U-No bar.
Fight with your hubby? Well, I'll tell you this truth:
You'll have no arguments with a Baby Ruth!
You feel so deprived, can't have that dessert?
Oh, a few secret little M&M's won't hurt!
If your fridge is dead or your washer won't start . . .
A Snickers or two will give you new heart.
So your toilet's run over. What do you say
That you go cuddle up with a Milky Way?
You feel so depressed and don't want it to linger?
Go have an affair with a Butterfinger!
There's just not one problem this world could evolve
That a trusty ol' Almond Joy couldn't solve.
Yes, those are the thoughts of fat in distress . . .
Of a ruined life . . . of a blubbery mess!
Those dirty rotten thoughts I will have no more,
'Cuz I want my body like it was before!

I want to bend over without having to grunt,
To take pictures . . . and not hold a baby in front!
To walk up some stairs and not gasp for breath,
To not lose ten years of my life . . . to death.
I want to be gorgeous and sexy and glad.
Not frumpy and fat and disgusting and mad.
I want to wear clothes and hats that would make
A handsome young man do a double take.
I want to be able to run through my house
And burn any stretch pants or maternity blouse.
And if Hershey's stock takes a terrible dive?
I don't care! 'Cuz at last, I'm comin' alive!
Let those who sell Twinkies be mad at me.
Who cares if they go broke? I'm gonna be *free*!
So no matter the trouble, no matter the strife—
This is the fattest day of the rest of my life!

DIARY
of a *Fat*
HOUSEWIFE

Prologue

The title of this book says it well. I am fat. I am a housewife. This is my diary. Right from the first word in my first entry, I intended to publish this diary one day. But when I started writing, I thought "one day" would be in about a year . . . when I became skinny. "Skinny" and "thin" are my way of saying "just right." I have no desire to become bony, but I would sure love to experience a flat tummy sometime in the twentieth century! After weighing more than 300 pounds, anything under 150 sounds "skinny" to me! Well, I'm not skinny yet, but I am at my lowest weight in ten years. And, fat or thin, I can wait no longer—it's time the world learned the truth about the misery of obesity.

You are about to begin a nine-year journey with me. You will discover what it is like to be fat . . . no, more than fat. As you read along with me, you will come close to experiencing morbid obesity. You will read about my significant triumphs and failures as a struggling dieter. Since I seldom wrote when I was feeling indifferent, many entries are volatile with emotion—either extreme despair or unearthly happiness. Sometimes I went for months without making an entry, so two consecutive entries may be a year apart and reflect crazily different moods.

During the past twenty years as an obese person, I have talked with hundreds of other fat people. They have shared many private thoughts and feelings with me about their weight. Though my highs may be more dramatic and my lows more depressing, I am certain that every fat person has experienced at some time a portion of the feelings I express in this diary.

My entries often deal only with food or seemingly ridiculous details of the number of pounds I'd lost or needed to lose by a specific date. If you are fat, you are already aware of how these thoughts dominate your thinking. (What a tragic waste of life!) If you've never had a weight problem, you'll grow to understand how fat people are hypnotized by food, mesmerized by weight-related numbers.

You also will begin to understand my philosophy regarding obesity. *I believe obesity is a disease.* Where food is concerned, something in my brain is not quite right. My upbringing encouraged and rewarded poor eating habits. It undoubtedly has had an impact on my continual craving for food. But I am convinced that these cravings are controllable, that my disease is manageable. I am ultimately responsible for the excess fat on my body. I blame nothing but myself.

It would be easy and convenient to believe many of the "fat philosophies" of today. They sound like a soothing balm to the soul who has suffered for years with excess poundage. Even though these philosophies are nothing more than lame excuses for further gluttony, the rotund are desperate to believe them. I wonder how many pounds of chocolate have been consumed while the fatty repeats:

1. This is the way I was meant to be. I have a low metabolism.
2. There is nothing I can do about my weight because everyone knows diets don't work.
3. My fat is my concern alone.
4. Big is beautiful.

Well, here is one fatty who adamantly refuses to be sucked into such unhealthy and foolish philosophies, tempting though they might be. I know such lines have been perpetrated and carefully massaged into our brains by the designers of fat clothing, the publishers of "big" magazines, and the promoters of other products that thrive on a fat population. I choose to rely on my own common sense, cultivated through twenty years of experience with morbid obesity, and respond to these statements with simple honesty:

1. People are not meant to eat until their bodies break out in ugly, hanging fat rolls. Hearts are not meant to suffer from the strain of pumping blood through hundreds of extra pounds of yellow, globby lard. *No matter what one's metabolism is, a person will lose weight if he takes in fewer calories than he expends.* Why is it that Americans have the highest rate of obesity? Because we eat too darn much! Think about it; there are no fat people in lands beset by famine.

2. The only sensible diet that *doesn't* work is the diet that *isn't* worked. I must swallow the bitter pill (instead of the chocolate) and accept the fact that I must be on a diet of some kind for the rest of my life.

3. Because your fat could cause you to die prematurely, leaving your spouse or children alone, *your fat is their concern.* Since your fat could cause you to suffer a stroke and become dependent on relatives for your care, *your fat is their concern.* If your fat keeps you out of swimming pools, off amusement park rides, or off the dance floor, leaving your family deprived of your company, *your fat is their concern.* Since your fat causes higher health insurance premiums for the general population, *your fat is everyone's concern*!

4. Big is beautiful? Over $33 billion were spent on weight-loss products and programs in 1990. I have yet to hear one advertisement on how to increase the size of your fat rolls or multiply the number of your chins! Nope! Nobody spends money to get fatter. Why? Because it's

ugly! (You can read more about the "Big Is Beautiful" myth in my diary.)

Throughout my diary, I frequently mention my childhood family and the experiences we've shared. I am one of nine children. I was born in 1952, before the time when such terms as *eating disorder*, *food addiction*, *high cholesterol*, and *fat-free* were part of our everyday language. My parents were overweight. They did not teach us healthy eating habits. They simply didn't know any better.

Ours was a poor family; my father lacked even a high-school education. We seldom had fresh fruit in the house, yet somehow we always had the money for candy, pastries, or ice cream. Our daily eating practices taught us to eat it now and eat it fast . . . or miss out on our full share.

Our upbringing had an adverse effect on our self-control. Both my parents and all my siblings are or have been fat. In fact, most of us have been dangerously obese. Most of my siblings have been addicted to alcohol, tobacco, and/or drugs. It's a good thing I have never touched any of those substances. I'd probably be the worst offender of all because at one time I was the fattest sibling of all.

Yet, as a child, I adamantly told myself I would *never* get fat. I'd grown up surrounded by it and swore I would never put myself in that mold. Ha! I *broke* the mold! Be warned: If you are old enough to read this book, you are old enough to be concerned about your eating habits. Don't fall into the depths of hell as I have. Protect yourself by establishing good eating habits now. Regardless of your age, reading my diary may help you avoid obesity later in life. It may even save your life, or that of a loved one.

In these pages, you will come to know my parents, my siblings, my husband, my children, and some of my friends. Some names and identities have been changed to protect . . . the guilty! For convenience and readability, I frequently interchange the pronouns *he* and *she*, as well as *him* and *her*. (There are many fat people of both sexes.)

I married at the tender age of eighteen to Allen, who is twelve years older than I. Our marriage has had as many ups and downs as my weight, but true love has prevailed. We have been blessed with six children. Each pregnancy, except the last, resulted in more hard-to-get-rid-of fat:

Jeremy, born September 23, 1972 (*68*-pound gain)
Jennifer, born September 23, 1975 (another *28*-pound gain)
Matthew, born September 7, 1977 (add *7* more pounds)
Tiffany, born August 11, 1981 (an additional *30* pounds)
Tyler, born August 10, 1986 (Yikes! another *34* pounds)

Yup, folks, I rolled into that hospital to deliver my fifth baby weighing well over 300 pounds! (A cumulative weight gain of 167 pounds!)

In the course of writing my diary, I have developed a weight-loss program that works for me. I call it my *Winning At Thinning* Action Plan.™ It's no magic formula for weight control; none exists. It's hard work to lose weight. It requires concentrated effort and sometimes superhuman willpower. But my *Winning At Thinning* Action Plan ™ seems to be a booster locomotive constantly behind me, pushing me up the steep diet track with an ever encouraging "I-know-you-can, I-know-you-can." It works! Whenever I use it, I lose it.

When I became pregnant with my last child, I had already dropped over 120 pounds. My Action Plan helped me keep my weight under control even while pregnant. Steven was born April 1, 1993. My acceptable, thirty-pound weight gain with him is already a thing of the past!

Reading and rereading my diary gives me the motivation to keep trying. It helps me remember—to almost relive— the acute agony of morbid obesity. I am determined never again to walk that hideous path. As I've reread my diary and edited it to prepare for publication, I have occasionally added notes to myself or to the reader, updating or clarifying some points.

Reading my diary also recalls the wonderful, invigorating

days of being in control of everything I put into my mouth, of being in control of me. The struggle to gain mastery over self is what this diary is all about.

Sunday, July 25, 1982

Ahhhh! Is this it? Can it really be? Have I made the ultimate commitment by putting pen to paper? Am I admitting to myself that I am finally ready? Why, the noise of my pen etching out these little marks on paper is nearly deafening! The noise, the deep breathing, the inner turmoil, the struggle—gasp—can I, will I spell out the final commitment? *I am going on a diet!*

Deep breath. There! I said it! Now you know. I am going on a diet, and you may come with me. If you are fat (not "plump" or "chubby"—I said *fat*!), maybe reading this will help you realize that you're not alone. Other fat people are experiencing similar frustrations and misery.

If you're not fat; if you don't own a pair of stretch pants or a maternity blouse; if your closet isn't full of clothes that fit you ten, twenty, thirty pounds ago; if you can still touch your toes, or even look down and *see* your toes, then you'd better come along for the insight. Find out what bizarre craving drove that fat lady to order her second banana split, why that obese man brazenly devoured a whole bag of potato chips in front of everyone.

Come with me—crawl inside for a while (I could easily

hold two or three)—and see what it's like. If you read with your heart, I promise that you will never despise or condemn fat people again. You'll develop an understanding and empathy for them. You'll discover the devastating tragedy of obesity.

There are a million and one reasons to diet, but the straw that broke this camel's back came yesterday. I walked into Allen's study. After our usual kissie-poo, I told him I craved his body. (Aren't I lucky? Even after eleven years of marriage, he still turns me on.) He said, "Now, that's a coincidence. Today I looked at some pictures I took of you in Tahiti ten years ago and lusted after your body!"

"Did you really?"

"Yes! You were *gorgeous!*"

Right then, something clicked in my brain . . . and broke in my heart. "You *were* gorgeous!" I heard it echo again and again in my head.

He wasn't being cruel. He hadn't meant to hurt me. But in that instant, ten years of fat misery seemed to slap me in the face. I was devastated by what I had done, for the obese human I had become.

I've decided to use this diary as a progress report, a place to vent my frustrations, disappointments, hurts, and hopefully my successes and joys. I love to write. Someday these pages will become a full-length book. I will call it *Diary of a Fat Housewife.* I can write it only one day at a time. That's how a diet works—one day at a time.

Tuesday, June 7, 1983

Well, well, well—fancy meeting me again. Notice the date? Yes, folks . . . ten and a half months later. My intentions last July were so earnest! I proved my sincerity by writing down in black and white, "I am going on a diet!" That's a major commitment. I should have written in my diary at the end of that first day. Writing in my diary will give me that added motivation to finally do something about dieting. So

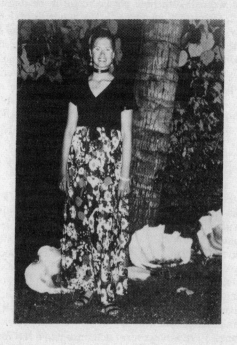

January 1972, 142 pounds. Yes, I was gorgeous. I remember loving to show off my long, slender neck.

write I must! (Oh! My stomach growled, first time in months! I'm so proud.)

I have written a motto for myself: "Today is the fattest day of the rest of my life." Tomorrow will be better . . . because I will be thinner.

I'm looking forward to getting up and weighing in. Hmmmm—wonder if I'll ever have the courage to write down how much I weigh. Silly as it seems, it's an unwritten rule that we certified fatties cannot, must not, divulge our weight.

It's as if we will somehow not be so fat if we don't admit our exact, disgusting poundage. In the hundreds of conversations I've had with other obese women, not once has anyone "told all." Even though we acknowledge we are fat, we tippy-toe around the issue of exact weight. We joke about ourselves. We share "fat" experiences. But we never, never ask each other the dreaded question: "How much do you weigh?" And we never tell the obvious truth, the truth that is written all over our faces (and all over our bodies): "I weigh 'x' number of pounds."

Sunday, October 2, 1983

I don't think I've awakened one day of my fat life (I've had two lives—one thin and one fat!) without determining that *this* was the day. This day, I would positively start my diet. Firm conviction. That firm conviction would last only until I reached the kitchen, where some stray cookie, leftover cake, or scoop of ice cream would tempt me for a full three seconds . . . and then I would succumb. Then hate myself desperately for eating it, probably not enjoying one crumb. Oh, come on, is that behavior seriously possible? Tragically, it's been ten years possible!

On June 7, 1983, however, I demonstrated a serious intent to diet. I made a calendar on which I wrote my weight: 257 pounds. (There! It's in print; I was a 257-pound lardo!) I also calculated the day I would be my ideal weight: 125 pounds. Yikes! I needed to lose 132 pounds. What a depressing thought! I had to lose more of me than I wanted to keep!

Just prior to June 7, I lost five pounds, taking me from 262 pounds down to 257. Compared to 132 pounds, a measly 5-pound loss sounds almost too ridiculous to mention—if you've never been fat. But I call attention to it here because that five pounds can have a negative psychological impact on the extremely obese person. It's a five-pound leeway to eat! You see, you can easily have a candy bar or bake a batch of cookies "for the family" (who are we kidding?) because you are down five pounds. If you pick up a pound or two, you'll still be down a pound or two from where you were. And no one will notice.

Brother! Do you realize how pathetic that last sentence is? "No one will notice" is the all-important consideration. I mean, you can eat like a pig for days, be sick to your stomach constantly from eating too much garbage, be too big for your seat belt, be unable to tie your own shoes or play on the floor with your children, be out of breath after climbing one flight of stairs, be signing your own death warrant by abusing your poor little heart and clogging your skinny little arteries . . . but heaven forbid someone should "notice" you've gained two pounds!

The day I made my calendar was important because it was my second step of commitment. The first step was starting a diary. Though I waited ten and a half months to make a second entry, it *was* the beginning. I am about to change my life, and keeping this diary is an important part of the plan.

I need to put my plan of attack in writing . . . and then read it regularly.

> *January 31, 1991. I firmly believe that the only way mortals can overcome serious sins or addictions is with the help of God, no matter what God is called or how God is visualized. Just as Alcoholics Anonymous acknowledges the need for help from a higher power, so must the foodaholic.*

These elements are necessary for my success:

1. Personal prayer
2. Scripture study
3. Diary entry
4. Weight-loss calendar
5. Exercise
6. List of foods to eat each day
7. Record of all food eaten
8. Time out to think thin

I started dieting again on September 14. I was perfect for nine days, didn't even lick my fingers. But September 23 marked the eleventh and eighth birthdays of my first two children. Cakes, candy, goodies galore! Just as tiny worms can creep in and destroy a whole beautiful apple, tiny little actions can creep in and destroy the most carefully conceived plan!

The next afternoon, on Saturday the twenty-fourth, I was watching TV. I had just survived a slumber party with twenty-three eight-year-old girls and felt I deserved a break. Suddenly, out of the blue, I could see in my mind that leftover birthday cake sitting on the kitchen counter. Just sitting there. I lost it! I ran to the kitchen, tore off a piece of cake, grabbed a large spoonful of chocolate frosting, and sneaked back to my bedroom to enjoy it. Even though the cake was pathetically mediocre, I downed the whole piece.

Now for the truly disgusting part. My appetite whetted, I rushed downstairs searching for a piece of candy—any candy—that the girls might have overlooked during their "treasure hunt" the night before. There were still four girls playing downstairs. I was humiliated. I hated myself. I wanted to die. Yet I proceeded to turn up couch cushions, look under chairs, move furniture. Of course, they asked what I was doing. So, I (gasp) lied. We fatties are professionals at lying. Do you think I could ever admit stealing from my little children's Halloween candy or Easter baskets? I tell myself I'll only "borrow" some, then buy replacement candy. But after replacing the replacement candy three or four times, I usually give up!

Yup, I looked those girls straight in the eyes and lied, "I need to find my barrette. I had it on last night and must have lost it down here." I was especially ashamed for lying to my own daughter. But I kept searching. Luckily, I didn't find any candy. There had been twenty-three girls looking for the hidden-candy treasure; how could I expect to find one single piece? I went so far as to ransack the bags the girls had filled the night before. I was going to take (okay, steal) an Almond

Joy from anyone's bag . . . but I couldn't find one dumb little Almond Joy in the whole house.

My chocolate fit died, drowned by my own disgust, and I made it through the day. Each day thereafter, I took a few forbidden bites. One night, I took my mom to the movies. She generously sent home a big bag of M&M's for the children. I accepted it for them. For the children? Get real! The second Mom was out of eyesight, I ripped that package open. I ate half the bag on the short drive home and ended up sick that night. When will I ever learn? I guess it sounds stupid to say I felt some pride because I didn't eat the whole bag. Yeah, it does sound stupid. I knew good and well that my mom would ask the children how they liked the treat she sent home to them, so I *had* to save some.

This morning, I forced myself to write in my diary to keep me from straying further. There are many more phases of my diet plan to get started on. Each day, I'm going to take the time to follow my plan of attack. I have discovered that I must put my duties as mother and wife second—behind my responsibility to me. It's imperative that I put me first, or else I will never be the wife and mother I am capable of being.

Thursday, October 6, 1983
246 pounds

Sunday, after I wrote that lengthy, motivating entry, I proceeded to cram my mouth full of garbage for the rest of the day. But wait, there's hope. Monday, Tuesday, and Wednesday I was perfect! Then—who knows why?—today I bonked out and ate like moths through wool.

I want to analyze it. I need to analyze it. I *must* analyze it. I cannot continue to repeat that same ridiculous behavior. Here I am, dying to be thin. I think of it every waking hour. Yet whenever I become upset, I eat. As if one more roll around my middle will alleviate some of my misery.

I'm depressed for several reasons. I haven't lost any weight for four days, yet I've been unusually good on my diet. I've been doing some minor remodeling on my kitchen, but it's still a pit, and I can't see an end to it. Although my children are terrific in most ways, right now they are being turkeys about keeping their bathrooms and bedrooms clean, and it's driving me crazy.

Of course, I set the perfect example of a spotless bedroom. Ha! I have to kick stuff out of the way to get to my bed! Which brings me back to the vicious cycle of obesity. I'm fat, my energy level is low, it's physically hard to move around, to climb stairs, to bend over. So my house is messy; the children learn from my pathetic example and add to the disorder. I get more and more depressed staying home all day in a messy house. So . . . I . . . eat! Okay, analysis over.

Tonight, I'm going to get my exerciser out of the closet, where it's lived for four years. (That's the stupid story of my life; my exerciser has been in my closet for four years. Think about *that!*) I'll put it in my bedroom and enjoy TV while I exercise. That is step three of my diet plan: exercise, exercise, exercise. (Step one is diary, step two is weight-loss calendar with goals, step three is exercise.)

Tonight I exercise. Tomorrow I eat only meat, eggs, vegetables, grapefruit, oranges, and apples. *Tonight*, too! I must start dieting from this moment; if I wait till tomorrow, I'll be fat forever.

That reminds me of a poem I once recited while lecturing to a group of women. The last lines read:

> I'm starting my diet, tomorrow, that's right . . .
> So let's have that last bite of pizza tonight!

"And exactly what were you lecturing on, Rosemary?" Why, weight loss, of course. At the time, I had just lost 65 pounds, weighed 150, and looked pret-ty fine. Today, at 246 pounds, I cringe with humiliation every time I see anyone who was present at one of my lectures. Needless to say, I haven't been asked to speak on that particular topic for quite some time.

Wow! Boy-oh-boy-oh-boy! I was through writing for the day, then I viewed a most distressing report about overweight children on *20/20*! I am compelled to record my feelings about it. This program discussed the problems, depressions, hurts, aches, and general misery of fat children. It showed fat farms—summer camps for fat children—which cost around $3,000 to attend! Some children were back for the fifth year in a row! Brother, what a pathetic society! But what really shook me was an interview with two of the mothers. The camera showed only their faces, but guess what? It was obvious that both mothers were grossly overweight.

Zap! Did I get the message: Fat moms produce fat children. Oh, no! No! I don't want to do that to my beautiful, precious babies. If I start dieting immediately, only Jeremy will remember my being fat, and he will have a hard time without pictures. I'm going to do it—for me and for them. Oh please, please, dear God . . . help me to help them. I never want them to go through this hellish experience—*never!*

Thursday, October 27, 1983
246 pounds

Oh, brother! I cannot believe myself! I lost seventeen pounds, then bingo! I went berserk! Over three weeks of crazy eating. I had tons of goodies and megasandwiches (oh, how I love them!), with lots of mayonnaise on fresh, soft bread. You know the kind of sandwich I speak of: stacked high, loaded with meat, cheese, cream cheese, sour cream, and anything else to add to the yumminess—and calories! But, miracle of miracles, in spite of all that, and macaroni and cheese and noodles, and let's throw in a little ice cream, I did show a small amount of self-control. I didn't gain any weight back.

Can you believe I was able to consume all that and still

maintain—not gain—weight? It is hard work; it requires nearly constant chewing to stay this fat!

Thursday, November 3, 1983
238 pounds

Monday was Halloween, a frightful day to resume dieting. I had eaten only an apple and a little beef jerky. Suddenly, shortly before going to bed, the old time bomb exploded! Within two minutes, I had stuffed into my mouth a piece of chocolate zucchini bread and three of my baby's candy bars. Yup, I stole from my two-year-old's Halloween candy. Unbelievable! At least I had enough sense to quickly leave the kitchen.

The next day, I was great, except for a momentary, crazy three seconds when I stuffed another piece of chocolate zucchini bread into my mouth. I almost choked on it! Yet I already knew from eating a piece the night before that I didn't like it! You figure it!

Like a breath of fresh air, yesterday I was perfect. I'm going to do it! I feel superhigh. Even though yesterday was the pits emotionally, I didn't eat one forbidden thing. I'm trying to make myself consciously think, "Why? Why should I let anger, hurt, or frustration drive me to eat?"

Today I weighed in at 238! Wonderful! Yet disgusting because I still have 113 pounds to go. But at least I want to *keep* more of me than I want to lose. I'm ecstatic. If I could only put feeling into words, why this very paper would become a song or a flower and dance around like a spirited nymph or fairy.

To think that next summer I can swim with my family, I can run races with my children, I can participate in sports, I can climb stairs, I can bend over. Why, I can even raise my husband's eyebrows again! Oh, the million and one things I'll be able to do!

Saturday, November 5, 1983
234 pounds

Oh, I am on, on, on! Do you know what this means? I want to fly out of my body and zoom around the world. I'm on my way to skinny. I'm escaping the vicious cycle.

Tonight, I was planning to go out to dinner with Allen, but Matthew, age six, performed surgery on himself. In reality, it was only a small cut on his finger. But from the looks of the bathroom where I found him, it appeared as if someone had cut his jugular vein! There was blood splattered on both sides of the room, from floor to ceiling. There was blood all over the floor and all over Matt, who was sitting on the bathroom counter. Blood covered the sink next to him. The diaper he used to clean up the blood was completely red!

Matt had simply cut his finger while trying to slice off the stem of a carrot. Instead of applying pressure to stop the bleeding, he kept shaking his hand. In the process of cleaning up, we found tiny pieces of chewed-up carrot on the bathroom counter beside him.

Allen: "Matt, what is this from?"

Matt: "From the carrot."

Allen: "You were eating your carrot in here after you cut yourself?"

Matt: "Well, I was bleeding with my right hand and eating with my left!"

Ah, the gems that come from children.

We didn't go out to dinner because it took us over an hour to clean up that mess. It was past ten-thirty, and I was too tired! What? Me too tired to eat? I tell you, I'm going to do it; this time I'm going to succeed!

The future is brighter as I see a thinner face staring back from the mirror. I want Allen to enjoy my feminine shape again! It's been a long, fat time.

Monday, November 7, 1983
232½ pounds

I ate four tiny candy bars and a big piece of cake last night. Why? All I can say is that another one of those ridiculous time bombs exploded! As I was setting the kitchen table last night, I suddenly knew I was about to eat a piece of cake; I knew it! The instant that first, wretched thought of cake entered my mind, I should have told Allen, "I hear the bomb ticking. Help me tonight. Stay with me. Keep me out of the kitchen!" But no. I didn't protect myself from me.

Get this: While the family was at the kitchen table waiting for me to put on the hot food, I actually put a piece of cake on a plate and sneaked it out of the kitchen into the dining room. When Allen asked, "Where are you going?" I answered casually, but with my heart racing, all the while embarrassed and ashamed, "Oh, I'm putting something away." Ahhhh! He fell for it! I left the cake on the dining room table and walked back into the kitchen.

I kept a sharp eye on the dog, who might decide to run into the dining room, jump up on a chair, and eat my carefully smuggled cake! In a few minutes, I sarcastically asked if it was okay if I left to use the bathroom. Allen smiled, and the children laughed, just as I had hoped they would. The sarcasm worked; they all fell for it.

So I left the kitchen, grabbed my plate off the dining room table, locked myself in the bathroom, and ate that tasteless, dry, store-bought cake covered with greasy frosting. I didn't enjoy one bite. It wasn't a pretty picture: I was sitting on the only chair in the room, the toilet. I was stuffing my mouth because I didn't have much time. And I couldn't help staring at myself as I took each bite because there was a huge, wall-to-wall mirror directly in front of me. Yet I ate the whole piece.

Thursday, November 17, 1983
233 pounds

Ten days later! I started each day with good intentions. I struggled to keep control of my ever-bending elbow. Then, as if some evil magician cast a wicked spell on me, the ol' brain would snap again.

One day, I was cooking treats for my daughter Jennifer's baptism reception. I had determined not to touch one bite of those luscious desserts. But suddenly I found myself chomping down on a mouthful of sugary, high-fat calories. And when I take that first bite of anything sweet—look out! I started *shoveling* things into my mouth. I went berserk. Finally, I was smart enough and brave enough to leave the kitchen. I knew I didn't have a chance in there.

I became sick that night, feeling as if I were going to throw up. When I woke up the next morning, I was sure I had learned my lesson, so I wasn't worried about overeating again. It wouldn't be worth it to go through another night of total discomfort! Even though I had to cook some more yummies that day, I was sure I'd be in control. I controlled myself all right—all the way to the kitchen!

I also ate too much Saturday, while serving the food at the reception. Sunday, I was afraid to weigh myself. So I pulled a typical, stupid, self-defeating "fat-person" trick: I ate a whole lot more. Monday, I felt positive I'd be good on my diet. I weighed in because I felt brave enough to face the music. My fears were a reality. I'd gained two pounds. Oh, gag, I weighed 235 again. Then, despite my actual terror of climbing back up the hell scale, I overate again. As all fat people know, "fatophobia" can almost keep you from breathing normally at this point.

Sure enough, Tuesday was two more pounds—I had reached a petite 237! And now I was on a hot run, because Wednesday I was 238. Panic, terror, what will I do, where will I go? How can I grab on to that "magic ring" and get off this horrible ride? *I can't think of anything but food, yet*

I don't want *to eat anything.* Oh please, God, help me make it through this one day.

I do pretty well during the day; then it seems toward evening, something bites me and shakes its ugly head from side to side till I feel like diving into a bowl of whipped cream. I'm writing to calm myself. I can't stand my body at this point. It has to get better.

Wednesday, November 23, 1983
235 pounds

Not only am I out of control in my eating, I am out of control with my temper. I scream at my children, at Allen, at anyone or anything that crosses my path. Total disgust for myself makes me impossible to live with. I blame anyone and anything, as long as it gives me an excuse to eat.

Three weeks from today, I'm leaving on a weekend trip to Canada with a bunch of skinny, beautiful young women— the New Oregon Singers, a group to which I once belonged. Depression time! I must earnestly dedicate myself to dieting and exercise for three weeks . . . and pray for a miracle.

I can do it. I *can* control me. Yet sometimes the craving for a chocolate candy bar is so strong, I can think of nothing else. It has to be something like the feeling experienced by the desert-stranded person who is craving a drink of water. It totally inundates me. Sometimes I audibly scream out, "NOOOO! I don't want any sweets. I want to be thin!"

Sunday, November 27, 1983
237 pounds

The terror is overwhelming. The misery is acute. I've been popping anything and everything into my mouth. And I . . . can't . . . seem . . . to stop! I must make it happen today.

Somehow! This must be it. Why do I eat when *I don't like it* and *I don't want to*?

When I was a member of the New Oregon Singers, Allen was their drummer. I'm not much of a singer, but I did meet the most important requirement to stand front row, center: great legs! Last week, Allen was asked to accompany the group to Canada because their current drummer can't make the trip. I was invited to travel with Allen, but, needless to say, I wasn't invited to sing with them—my legs aren't that great at the moment!

So now I have seventeen short days to lose 100 pounds! All the females on that trip will be skinny. As the day comes closer, the pressure intensifies. The horror takes my breath away. I can't possibly go looking like this. It's sheer hell! If I miraculously lost 20 pounds, I'd still weigh in at 217. Yikes! That's a baby whale.

I keep imagining myself on the bus with all those skinny bodies. The contempt in their eyes, the disgust on their faces, their barbed words. So I've had four children. That's no excuse! Some of those pencil-thin women have had babies, too. They can't see any of my good qualities. They are hidden somewhere in these ripples of blubber.

In six months, I could be a new person. I could run, swing, slide, swim, play tennis, ride a bike, do all those things I'm too fat for at present. It can be revolting to see a fat person participate in those activities, but fat does not destroy the desire to do them. I still want to have fun. Do you think fat cuts out all memories of those wonderful, "skinny" activities? Do you think fat dissolves the desire and need for physical exercise? No! Sometimes I feel my body aching with the desire to *move*! To dance—I mean, really dance!

Do you have even a sparkle of an idea of how much I long to exercise my body? I lie in bed, going over each glorious move, as I do curl-ups, leg lifts, jumping jacks—in my mind. I relive the invigorating sensation my body had when I exercised as a thin person. But it's all in my imagination while I lie in my bed! Insanity? Yes—and part of the paralysis that occurs with fat people. Movement takes extraordinary effort;

it's easier just to sit and think about it, to remember doing it. And while you're sitting there, habit sets in, making it doubly hard to ever break free of the "sofa slug syndrome."

My blood is starting to boil! I'm not going to be a fat-person fool. I'm going to *spend* the rest of my life, not throw it away! I'm going to get up, *now*, and have that glorious feeling of invigoration I used to have. I'm going to exercise! I'm going to do fifty jumps on my minitramp. But first, I have to remove the ton of clutter that has been dumped on it. Yup, it's just like me to have my exercise equipment covered with junk. Oh, what a fool I am!

January 28, 1991. I never went on that dumb trip with the skinny singers. I was too humiliated to go. Allen and I had several horrible fights shortly before the scheduled departure. I finally realized I was deliberately picking fights because I was so paranoid about going. I was desperate; I had to do something. I determined to protect myself. I was thinking of Allen, too. I told him I couldn't do it. I didn't want to mortify both of us by going on that trip. When I made that decision, the pressure burst like a taut balloon, and I ate like there was no tomorrow.

Allen went without me, taking six-year-old Matthew instead. Once again, the disease of obesity had struck. Fat rolls had done their dirty work. Once again, I had lost my freedom to chocolate bars, my self-made god.

Friday, March 16, 1984
243 pounds

Up to 243 again! I'm feeling desperate. I'm going crazy. I'm going to die. I can't be seen in public. I'm a disgusting, despicable example of womanhood. I cannot go on living. I do not *want* to go on living, not like this. It's not real living, anyway. I must either quit eating like a maniac or find a way to end it all. Suicide! There . . . I said it; I said the ugly word, at last. I admit it; I do think about it. Sometimes the only thing that keeps me from suicide is the thought of someone trying to lift me into a coffin. And what if I couldn't fit? I do not write one word of this entry with a smile on my face. I am *deadly* serious. I have a critical decision to make. Is food more important to me than life itself? I don't think it is, but I live as if it is. Oh, the aching, almost painful longing I have to be in control of me. I do not want to play this game anymore.

Saturday, April 28, 1984
242 pounds

Have experienced one and a half months of hell since my last entry. Can remember the desperation as I wrote. What is it that influences a person to start overeating again? I wonder if there is some sort of brain surgery possible to correct the "little impulses" that drive a person almost uncontrollably to *eat*.

How can I do this to me? How can I totally deform my once delectable body—over Twinkies, cheesecake, ice cream, chocolate candy, and strawberry mousse? By what possible rationale? It's beyond belief. No sane person would do it. Why me? No more, I've had enough.

The sheer hell of these past few months is incomprehensible. I think of prisoners being tortured by the Nazis. How horrible that one person should inflict torture on another. Yet I am daily, hourly, by the minute, torturing myself. How pathetic!

Many times every day I walk down the hall to my bedroom. At the end of the hall is a full-length mirror. My eyes, like a magnet, are drawn to my distorted figure. I look like a balloon with a ball on top, somehow walking on stilts (my legs are relatively thin). I look like I'm thirteen months pregnant.

Every time I sit down, I feel the rolls of my stomach hanging in my lap. These last fifteen pounds have made a difference—a *huge* difference. My fat rolls have become so much larger that I can't rest my arms in front of me, because there's no place to rest them!

With every step I take, my body betrays me and yells to the world, "Hear how her legs rub together? Hear her ham hocks?" Every time I put my arms at my side, I feel the hips, hips, hips! Every time I look down, my body screams out, "Feel your triple chin!" How I hate my disloyal body!

I am aware of my obesity every minute—*every minute*. This must surely be akin to hell. Sorrow, pure misery, over something that need not be. No one forces me to eat, no one ties me down, opens my mouth, and pours in chocolate. Only me! I have caused my own suffering, and that greatly intensifies the whole problem of obesity. My weight is my own fat fault! What a vicious circle.

A few days ago, I was visiting with three friends. Two of us were obese, a third was not quite as heavy, and the fourth is constantly struggling to maintain her relatively thin figure. The thin one told this story:

"Yesterday I opened and ate a whole package of cookies that I had bought with my husband the night before. He came home from work unexpectedly early and, much to my chagrin, started looking for the cookies we'd bought. When he asked where they were, I laughed, 'Oh, I've hidden them.' He insisted on looking until he found them, so I said, a little more emphatically, 'You'll never find them; I've *really* hidden them' (. . . in my stomach!). Then, I nonchalantly told my husband I needed to run to the store to buy something for dinner. I asked him to watch the kids. Whew, I bought an identical package of cookies to replace the ones I'd eaten, so he never knew."

Okay, people, can you relate? If you can't understand or comprehend this behavior, you are blessed beyond belief. Remember this: the story is true. And the guilty party was thin. Thin, do you hear me? Think of the additional finagling those of us who are fat go through! The lies, the tricks, the deceit, the hiding and destroying of evidence. And worse yet, the destroying of lives.

The conversation at my friend's house continued. We discussed diets, fat, poundage—I mean, we talked blubber!

As I sat there, I felt as if I were on the outside looking in. I was thinking, "Here we are, four grown women. We are all having a hideous time in life fighting our own fat selves. Our problem is totally self-induced. It devastates our ability to function, to enjoy life. These women need something more concrete than any weight program on the market. They need my plan. I *must* do it. I must implement my program. Yes, it is more than a plan, it is actually a program for success! I have something to offer the fat people—especially women— of the world."

My desire to lose weight, keep a diary, and then use it to help others, set itself in concrete that afternoon.

Thursday, May 3, 1984
243 pounds

Another story for *That's Incredible*! Monday night, to my horror and delight, I spied a half-package of M&M's tucked into an Easter basket. Pop, pop, pop, three M&M's were in my mouth, followed by the rest of the pack. Ah, the flavor, the comfortingly familiar sensation. In fact, it was so nice to "visit" this old friend, I couldn't wait till the next day, when I could buy some more. Can you believe this? Selling my soul—well, at least my happiness—for a few lousy M&M's, a few chocolate-coated poison pellets!

Wednesday, May 9, 1984
243 pounds

Did I do it? Did I oink out? Do dogs have fleas? Does chocolate have calories? Yes, yes, yes, and yes! Disgusting, horrible, despicable. But in minor defense: It's been only six days since my last entry. At least I didn't wait one or two years to try again.

This time, I'll do it. This time is different. This time, I will succeed because I've implemented step four. I'm writing down a list of exactly what I *will* eat. I've found I can deceive myself into eating any food, maneuver my own conscience into agreeing with me that a luscious chocolate dessert is, after all, made with milk, and "everybody needs milk!" I am professional at this game, I can rationalize ingesting *anything*!

I'll stop stating what I *won't* eat (negative approach) and start declaring the food I *will* eat (positive approach). Positive is always better than negative! And as accomplished people know, to attain any important deed, it is essential to have goals, written goals. So I will write down my intended menu. Seeing it in black and white will make me much more committed.

Yesterday, after a horrid morning of overeating, I had a talk with Allen. We decided that, daily, I would tell him what I will eat. We will write it down, and I will report each night. Another critically important concept: Report regularly on your success (or failure) to a trusted person. It is a winner's principle. It is invaluable insurance toward achieving your goals!

Saturday, September 22, 1984
250 pounds

Four months without writing a word. Who would ever believe it? Why should anyone else when I can't myself? Thank goodness I've written at least this many pages. They offer a clear-cut solution to obesity. This moment, I'm going to get up and follow the steps I've formulated. I'll report back to my diary as the last step.

Done! I can't write fast enough. Words are not sufficient to describe this sensation. This is it . . . I feel life again! What can I liken it to? A flower blooming; a baby bird opening its eyes for the first time; the final, awe-inspiring note of the "Hallelujah Chorus." I long to simply don jeans and a T-shirt and clean house without being hampered by 125 pounds of fat hanging on my body!

I weighed in at 250 pounds today, but I'm not going to get depressed. I'm just going to get going. Okay. I need more than a mental list of the steps I have developed. I need a written checklist I can follow each day. That's it! I will call it my Daily Checklist. My one hope. I'll do it immediately!

Tuesday, December 18, 1984
250 pounds

After reading my last entry, it is hard to comprehend that I am capable of so completely disappointing myself! On the other hand, after almost three more months of drastic failure, causing many suicidal thoughts, it's amazing to me that this human spirit has any hope left, still wants to try, try again. But I do! More than that, I have a conviction that I will yet walk this earth as a trim, lovely lady.

I wonder if I will ever be sure why I have been given this trial. I know that I must overcome it. If I don't, my body remains a visible-to-all-the-world sign that I am not in control of my life. Today is the first day of the rest of my life. Today is the *fattest* day of the rest of my life.

Friday, January 11, 1985
250 pounds

Writing that last entry inspired me to be good on my diet for a few days. But—don't fall off your chair with shock—I'm now cramming and chewing like Godzilla eating New York.

There are no words disgusting enough or full of enough self-loathing to adequately express this fat person's true feelings. "Living hell" barely scratches the surface. It barely begins to describe the real, gut-rending torture of walking into a room of pretty, thin ladies. Oh! Agony!

Today my sister Debbie called me. Her first words were, "Are you using your new exercise bike?" She proceeded to bemoan the eight pounds she's gained in the two months since she's been married. Then she vowed to lose those eight plus the twelve additional unwanted pounds she is carrying. How typical! Half my conversations are about weight. Everywhere I go, people are obese. The tragedy of it overwhelms me to the point of tears. All those people crying out for help! I want to get control of myself, and then I can help others.

I have many experiences to record. If only I could write all day . . . but a person *has* to eat. Ha! Ha! Today I will eat only: meat, eggs, grapefruit, and vegetables. I did it before, shortly after Jennifer was born. On that "grapefruit diet," I lost sixty-five ugly pounds in five months. I can do it again.

> *September 25, 1991. Okay, okay, okay. That was then, this is now. I do not advocate heavy consumption of meat and eggs in this enlightened age of fat and cholesterol awareness. Neither do I advocate other stupid fad diets. There are too many delicious, healthy alternatives!*

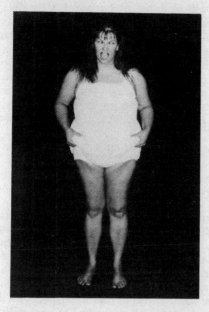

January, 1985, 260 pounds. Yikes! The expression on my face is exactly how I felt about me at this weight. (I still can't believe I let Allen take this picture!)

Wednesday, January 16, 1985
245 pounds

Some people look upon dieting as a deprivation. For me, it's a regaining of self-control. It's flying without a plane, without drugs. It's an ice skater doing a pirouette in the middle of the rink with 3 million pairs of eyes glued on her, and she keeps twirling. It's "the bombs bursting in air" on the Fourth of July. It's Christmas morning for a six-year-old. It's trick-or-treating, Easter bunny, Santa Claus, and Disneyland all rolled into one exquisite experience. It's the only possible thing that could make me feel this way!

Jeremy is twelve, in the seventh grade. I'm aware that he worships me in many ways. He's a darling, loving child. In the past, when I visited him at his elementary school, he was proud of me and happy to see me come. Last September, he transferred to a middle school—only sixth-, seventh-, and eighth-graders. I asked if he wanted me to join him for lunch sometime. He lowered his eyes; he hesitated answering me. "Well . . . "

"Jeremy, would you be embarrassed of me because I'm so fat?"

"Well . . . "

"Jeremy, it's okay. Let me put it this way: If I were thin, would you want me to visit you at school?"

"Oh, yeah!" he answered with much enthusiasm.

Well, folks, that's it in a nutshell! Re-al-i-ty. Fat is definitely not in! I ached in every fat cell of my body that minute.

Hang in there, Jeremy! I'm on my way. By the end of this school year, or next September at the latest, you'll be begging me to come and eat with you. You'll want to show me off to everyone you ever met in your whole life. You'll hope the "coolest" guy in the school thinks I'm your girlfriend!

Okay, so the girlfriend idea is a little farfetched—but you *will* want to show me off! No more cute little comments from your friends, like your fellow saxophone player. Upon seeing me for the first time, he commented, "That your mom? She's cute. A little chubby, but cute!" Chubby, my eye. Let's talk tub o' lard—blubber anonymous—fat city—bench breaker. I mean, we're talking 250 pounds here!

Oh, yes, I'm going to have a whole new life with my children—I'm going to have real, get-down-and-play-in-the-dirt-with-'em fun!

And talk about fun . . . could anything be more fun, more out-of-this-world desirable than to "slip into something a little more comfortable" for my husband? Something soft, silky, and—dare I say it?—sexy . . . and actually *look* sexy? How I crave to be desired. How I want my gorgeous, perfect-bodied, still-fits-into-his-army-uniform-after-twenty-years husband to embrace me and not be separated by a foot of fat stomach. I want him to run his hands down my back and not have them get stuck between rolls of blubber. I want him to be able to put his arms around my waist . . . and feel a waist. I want him to ask me to raise my dress a little so he can look at my gorgeous legs again, instead of being turned off by my fat knees. I'm tired of being twice the woman he married!

Yes, I want to be thin again for Allen and for my children, but most of all, for me. I want to find *me*! I'm not 245 pounds. I'm a thin person, trapped inside a fat body. I'm a Rose Festival princess! Surely there's a zipper somewhere. If I could just find the pull, and unzip this most unbecoming costume and step out as me—as I really am—like a butterfly emerging from its most unbecoming cocoon.

Thursday, January 17, 1985
243 pounds

Today will be better than yesterday because I'm two pounds lighter! If two pounds sounds like no big deal to you, try strapping a two-pound can of shortening on your arm or stomach or thigh for a day.

Yesterday I was surrounded by tons of temptation, but I didn't succumb. Right after I'd finished writing in my diary, my sister Rebecca called. She asked, "Can Tiffany come over and spend the night? Oh, and on the way, can you pick up a half pound of peanut M&M's for me, and I'll treat you to something, too?" I could surely relate to Rebecca's need for chocolate, but I knew that the high she'd get from eating it was nowhere near the high I'd get from resisting.

I am feeling so in control, so incredibly good, so—could it be?—righteous. Being in control is the quintessential high for someone who has been devastatingly out of control for twelve long years.

You can bet your last candy bar I didn't eat any peanut

M&M's! I marched into that store, picked up a half pound of those dirty little life-suckers, and marched right out again. Not for one tiny second did the thought of eating a candy bar enter my mind. It was astonishing!

Last night, after repairing some broken water pipes at my brother Jay's house, my dad offered to treat the three of us to something to eat. It was 11:00 P.M. "Sure," I said, then nonchalantly added, "I can have chicken or steak." (I said it as if I didn't pig out regularly on sweets and fast foods.) Dad suggested Burgerville USA. I could get a fish fillet there, and that would also be acceptable on my diet. Problem number one: they were out of fish fillets. Problem number two: they offered no diet drinks. Problem number three: the salad bar was closed for the night.

Did I succumb? Didn't I have the right to a hamburger? Dad and Jay were each getting a double cheeseburger; didn't I merit something? A few days ago, you can bet I would have scarfed down a double and a milk shake. But today? The new me? *No way, man!* "I'll have water, please." Was this Joan of Arc, or what? Again, I felt almost righteous sitting there sipping my noncaloric, healthy water!

Saturday, January 19, 1985
239 pounds

The fat person's mind behaves in a contradictory manner. It's amazingly complex. His purpose for eating is a million miles from survival. Instead of consuming food, he becomes consumed by the thought of food. Instead of eating to be filled, he eats to become *ful*filled. But since food cannot satisfy the need for fulfillment, he keeps searching—and eating—and searching and eating. Eating becomes tantamount to nirvana, yet it ironically leads to hell.

How many times have I stretched across my bed late at night with my carefully purchased hoard of precious candy bars? The children in bed, Allen at a church meeting or out playing drums with a dance band. The TV flicked on to whatever waste-of-time program happens to be airing. Excited over the five to ten delightful little bars of chocolate ecstasy before me, disgusted with myself for buying them. Crunching into a sensational Snickers bar; snickering at myself for thinking no one will notice. Munching a sickeningly rich Peanut Butter Cup, eyes shut, almost trembling with pleasure; hating every bite of it, knowing what it is doing to my body, as it munches away at my sex life, my whole life! Dissolving into the pure joy of an Almond Joy; knowing there will be *no* joy, only shame, with the last bite. Slowly popping those sure-to-do-no-harm little M&M's into my mouth, one or two at a time, letting them melt slowly away. Then the Butterfinger, the Twix, the Baby Ruth (almost justified because of the nutritional value of peanuts). All the while knowing how sick I will feel in the middle of the night from the inhuman amount of chocolate I've consumed in twenty short minutes.

The getting sick part happens all too often. I've wakened countless times in the middle of the night, feeling absolutely wretched. I have rushed to the bathroom, being afraid I was going to vomit, knowing full well the origin of the problem was ten candy bars. Sometimes I vomit. Sometimes I don't. I hate throwing up with a passion, so I pray, "Oh please, please, God. Please hear me this one last time. I have no right to ask for your help because I brought this on myself, knowing full well I could get this sick. But please help this horrid feeling to go away. I feel I might die [*I almost hope I will die at this point*]. I am embarrassed to ask, but if I have any chances left, please, please help me." I chew a couple of Rolaids, sip a little water, breathe deeply, and after twenty minutes to one hour, I can crawl back to bed and hate myself to sleep.

But no more! I'm on my diet, and I'm going to do it. The most remarkable thing about a diet is that it is, in reality, a way of repenting of the sin of overeating. It is visible evidence of a repentant soul. The marvelous experience of true repentance cannot sufficiently be described. It is uplifting to the highest level. It's a feeling I've tried to describe several times before—like flying. It's been years since I've felt this way.

> *February 9, 1991. The next time I am tempted to eat an excess amount of any sweets, I will read the above entry slowly and carefully. I will reread it— several times if necessary. I will remember being sick and nauseated instead of eating until I actually am.*

Sunday, January 20, 1985
240 pounds

I sure do relate to a joke I heard a comedian tell a few weeks ago: "Men! You can't live *with* 'em . . . and you can't shoot 'em!" Most of them (and I have one of the best) do deserve to be shot from time to time. I've been on my diet for one solid week, feeling as if I am finally repenting of twelve years of body abuse. It's a celestial experience.

Nevertheless, right this moment, I'm mad. For the first time in almost fourteen years of marriage, I've been up, emotionally supercharged for over a week. Yet Allen, who by nature is chipper, enthusiastic, and energetic 362 days out of the year, and who is thin and gorgeous 365 days yearly, called me a hypocrite tonight for being excited about my diet but still able to get upset with him for being late for dinner.

But you know what? I'm going to stay excited. I'm not going to use his mean and rotten words for an excuse to eat. In spite of him, I'm going to stay on my diet!

Monday, January 21, 1985
239 pounds

This dieting business has to be a twenty-four-hour-a-day commitment. It must be the first thing you think of upon waking and the last thing you mention at night. It must be your number one thought through the day. *It's hard work.* And it's critical to talk daily with someone who can give you support with your diet.

Last night I was angry with Allen. Result: no discussion with him about my diet. And today I overate at dinner, I didn't stick to my Daily Menu!

And wow! Did I ever lose it with my children. I lose control of my eating, and then I lose control of me. I want life to be better for them. I want them to learn to be in control of themselves so they will be *free*. Free from overeating. Free from alcohol and other drugs. Free from smoking, lying, and gambling. The best teacher is example, so I'm trying desperately to show them how I escaped—made my jailbreak, my leap for freedom!

Tuesday, January 22, 1985
240 pounds

I have written another motto for myself. I already tell myself, "This is the fattest day of the rest of my life." Today, when I was feverishly contemplating a second helping at dinner, even though I was full, this thought flashed into my mind: "Rosemary, stop and think. The less you eat, the more you lose!" Yes! The less I eat, the more I lose. I sat there and had a virtual stare-down with the remaining food. I kept repeating over and over, "The less I eat, the more I lose." It worked. I won. No seconds for me.

Even though I've been strict on my diet, I haven't lost any weight for four days. This is the point, that precarious, life-and-death, dangerous point where one says, "It's no use. See? I can't lose weight—even when I eat right!" and then flees to the store for a visit with a sweet old friend—or two . . . or ten. You finally make that magic button click on in your brain, and you diet till you lose that easy-to-come-off first ten pounds. But then your body adjusts to the new diet, and you get down to losing the solid, set-in-its-ways fat—and that's hard work, so you give up.

But this time, I have not succumbed. I am familiar with the sneaky trick my body pulls. If I diet faithfully for a month, I will lose around twenty pounds. Daily dieting is how you do it, but it's monthly dieting that shows results.

Yesterday I dropped in on my friend Pam. We are both extremely overweight. It was inevitable: We talked fat. From my twelve years of experience as a genuine, bona fide fat person, I can make the following statement accurately. Any time two fat female friends get together, they will have a conversation that includes some discussion of fat in general, new diet plans or fads, food they pigged out on, husbands' complaints about fat, how hard it is to find fat-lady clothes, *or* some yummy, new cookie recipe the other one positively must try.

This day was no exception:

Me: "How ya' doin'?"

Pam: "I've started going to Weight Watchers."

As we talked, it became glaringly apparent that the spouses of fat people need to better understand the fatty's plight. Spouses need to learn what they *can* do to help and what they absolutely, positively, no matter what the circumstances, must *never*, ever do!

I was happy that Pam had joined Weight Watchers. *Any* step a fat person takes toward a sensible diet plan is progress, a step in the right direction. Now, the Weight Watchers program is not for me. I couldn't sit there with 200 other fat ladies, analyzing each one, getting slightly hysterical till I could find one fatter than I. No, that's not my way. But I acknowledge that it *has* worked for many people.

I was happy that Pam had mustered up the courage it took to go to that first meeting. That is no small feat; I was proud of her. But I was outraged with her husband's response: "Why are you doing that, anyway? Why do you have to spend six dollars a week? Why don't you just quit eating?" Oh! He ought to be horsewhipped! Doesn't he know *any* of the pain, misery, and hell his wife has suffered these past six years? Doesn't he have a vague idea of the inner courage she displayed by attending a meeting for fat people? Doesn't he realize he could be her greatest help and hope? And his "just quit eating" comment is the all-time ignorant antidote for obesity. Yet thin people continually make that absurd statement, as if we fatties had never thought of lowering our intake!

Someone needs to start an organization to offer help and guidance to thin spouses of fat people. Spouses have an enormous potential as a catalyst in the recovery process. The world needs a list of rules for spouses of fat people. Pam has been fat for six years! Her husband should have been 100 percent encouraging. How *dare* he belittle her efforts? (They could easily afford the six dollars.)

Then—oh, horror of horrors—this uncaring husband looked at his wife and grumbled, "When's the last time you saw 200 pounds, anyway? I think it's gross when a wife outweighs her husband!" I heard my own sharp intake of breath. I felt like a mother bear whose cubs were being attacked! Was this man totally blind, deaf, and dumb? How could he be so openly degrading to his own wife? I wanted to smack him up side of the head till I knocked some sense into him. Those kinds of words, those ugly, cruel, stab-'em-in-the-back-and-twist-the-knife kinds of remarks frequently trigger the biggest eating binge you could ever dream of.

Oh, spouses, please realize you have within yourself the power to make or break the best-laid diet plans. The psychology of the fat person is totally bizarre. We are irrationally sensitive. We often make comments and decisions—then wait to see how you will react. And your reactions are all-important to us. When I tell you I'm going on a diet, I put out a million little feelers. It almost seems each little fat cell in my body has eyes and ears to detect your most minuscule response. If you raise your eyebrows a fraction of an inch, if your mouth even suggests a smile, if you grunt a "That's great" but have an "Oh, sure" in your eyes—I can tell. And I wait. If your response gives me the slightest reason, I'll think to myself,

"He doesn't care, anyway, so why should I? I'll show him who's fat!" Another contrived excuse to eat.

A simple, honest "Wow, honey! I know you can do it!" would mean everything in the world to me. Just *don't* laugh at me. Don't give up hope. Help me. Hope for me . . . for us. Pray with me . . . for me . . . for us. I can—we can—do it!

> *June 12, 1991. I have made a list of "Do's and Don'ts for Helping Your Spouse, Loved One, or Friend Conquer Her Disease of Obesity." It is in the Appendix. Read it, oh, so carefully, all you spouses of fatties out there. Read it, friends or relatives of fatties. There is much you can do. Don't leave your obese friend or family member to suffer alone. Obesity is a serious, life-threatening disease. Your fat friend needs help and support, just as your friend with cancer or diabetes does.*

Wednesday, January 23, 1985
238 pounds

Writing about Weight Watchers yesterday called to mind an experience I had in March of 1979. Dear Allen. Dear, caring-but-still-did-not-understand-my-weight-paranoias-after-being-married-to-me-eight-years Allen. He came home from work one night and announced that he was taking me on a surprise date.

We had a standing date every Friday night, but this was a weeknight. It was very romantic. Why, a surprise date was as exciting as receiving an unexpected bouquet of flowers or a box of fancy chocolates! (Naaah! It wasn't as monumental as getting chocolates.)

I couldn't pry a single, tiny clue from Allen. Even as we were driving, he wouldn't tell me where we were headed. My first indication of the evening of bliss that lay ahead came when Allen told me that this date was the result of something he had heard on the radio. At that moment, an apprehensive feeling started to creep over me. The longer we drove, the more intense grew my discomfort.

When we pulled into the parking lot at Kaiser Sunnyside Hospital, my apprehension escalated into serious paranoia. "Allen, I need to know right now exactly what this surprise date is." (I didn't like the looks of that hospital.)

I remember the scene well. We were parked in our little red Opel GT. The skies were clear. Stars were out. The trees were barely beginning to bud. Allen spoke softly. "I thought we could go to a meeting here." My heart raced. My apprehension, my paranoia, had been well founded. I knew before I asked, before he answered, what the real scenario was.

My mouth was dry, my lips felt heavy and hard to move. But I was finally able to utter, "What kind of meeting, Allen?" I was terrified of the answer I knew I would hear.

You ever heard the expression "pregnant pause"? Well, this pause was so pregnant, it was on the delivery table! Allen almost whispered, "It's an Overeaters Anonymous meeting."

I felt as if every vein, every blood vessel in my body, burst at that moment. A hot blackness exploded within me. "Take me home, Allen!" I don't think I screamed . . . yet. I remember being numb with humiliation, hatred of Allen, hatred of life, hatred of self. The numbness is a vivid memory. It's interesting how numbness can sort of slide into steel resolve. I guess because they are both so cold.

My resolve to "show Allen" at that point was unbelievably set. How *dare* he take me to a meeting for fat people without telling me? What did he think I would do, go up to the front and bear my testimony of chocolate? Did he think I would dance into that meeting with a smile on my face and a song on my lips and jump on the nearest scale in sight? Did he think I would sit there with my stomach bulging onto my lap and wish we could do this more often? Didn't he realize that going to a meeting like that took weeks of preparation, weeks of getting your mind set for the ordeal, weeks to *diet* for, for crying out loud? Oh, Allen, how could you put me through this agony, this degradation, this burning pain?

I don't remember how much of that I said out loud and how much I kept inside. Whatever I told Allen was only a fraction of the extreme depth of emotion I was feeling at the time. I'm not sure how much I yelled, screamed, or cried. But I am sure of one thing: Allen, dear, one-step-closer-to-understanding-my-weight-paranoia Allen, will never again take me to a surprise meeting for fat people—never, ever again!

Friday, January 25, 1985
240 pounds

Thank goodness for my diary. Thank goodness someone takes a little time to help and encourage me . . . even if it's only myself! From here on out, I'm going to stick to my Daily Menu like Sugar Babies stick to your teeth! I'm going to disappear, one greasy, ugly pound at a time.

I still weigh 240 pounds. Do you hear, Rosemary? Two hundred and forty pounds! You weigh more than most of the players on a college football team. Get a grip and lose a hip, girl!

Saturday, January 26, 1985
238 pounds

Oh, glorious morning. What an exhilarating, spine-tingling pleasure—238 pounds. The thirties. I'll never see the forties again. I feel like Charles Dickens' Scrooge when he awakened the morning after his visit from the three spirits. I'm eternally grateful I've "awakened" before I'm too old to appreciate it. Yes, I've lost some young, beautiful years, but the lessons of those years are invaluable to me.

There is no way one could understand or describe this literal hell-jail, these bars of fat I have built with my own hands, molded by my own choice. As I'm beginning to unlock the door, this exhilarating feeling of escape makes the misery almost worth it. I want to run out on my balcony and yell to all the world: "Life is grand, don't waste it. Live each second. Take advantage of each day. Take control of yourself, so all the joys of the world can be yours!"

Everyone should read *A Christmas Carol* once a year to appreciate the stupidity of some of our ways. Ebenezer Scrooge was a creature who lived in abject misery, by his own hand. When he finally came to his senses and changed his miserable ways, the heavens themselves seemed to open before him. He delighted in every little thing. He experienced the miracle of repentance—of changing his life for the better!

I have mutilated my once lovely body, and I have sorely, painfully, paid the price each waking moment. But, oh, the beauty of repentance, of changing my ways. Although I am still obviously a grotesque hunk of human flesh at 238 pounds, my attitude about myself is no longer one of pure hatred. Life no longer seems bleak and depressing. It's a pleasure, full of unlimited potential for happiness.

It is a tragedy that we mortals are capable of digging devastating pits for ourselves! My brother Jay is in one. A black, bottomless hole. Jay is an alcoholic. Just as he drinks out of control, I *eat* out of control, so my empathy for him is especially acute. Like myself, Jay is a miserable creature. He has slipped to the low rung on the ladder of hope. As his life is a mess, so also is his house. He is in a vicious cycle, all too familiar to me. Coming home to a messy house, he drinks to escape reality. I felt heroic the night I helped Jay clean his house. It made me realize how important it is to have my own life in a semblance of order so that I have time and energy to help others.

Besides their more obvious problems, many fat people deal

daily with another subtle addiction: television. What a time waster! And what do we fat people do while watching our favorite TV programs? We eat. Out of habit. There is no TV program on earth that is not 100 percent better with a bowl of ice cream, a giant-size candy bar, a package of cookies, or (D), all of the above.

If, by some miracle, you're currently dieting, be prepared, or the advertisements will get you. They will fill your brain so full of the mouthwatering delicacies that you won't have a chance. Your resolve will melt like a chocolate bar left on the dashboard on a hot day, and, one more time, you'll make the trek to the kitchen. . . .

Sunday, January 27, 1985
235 pounds

Even though Jeremy, my twelve-year-old son, broke his foot yesterday; even though my nine-year-old daughter has the flu; even though there's a six-foot hole in my front yard, as the repairman is trying to unearth a broken water pipe, I am excited about life! I weigh 235 pounds, 15 pounds less than I did two short weeks ago. I am going to do it! I feel much better! I *can't believe* the difference that a mere fifteen-pound loss has made in my ability to fit into clothes and to move around.

I can hardly wait to be able to button my winter coat all the way. It's ridiculous to be walking around in 20-degree weather with my coat gaping open a full six inches. I sometimes wear a scarf that hangs down and partially fills in the gap. It helps a little, but I look like a fat fool. Next time you wonder why that fat person never buttons his coat or suit when it's freezing outside, check it out. It probably can't reach across his extended middle. Oh, it's such a disgrace. Under those circumstances, only a fool would complain about the cold for fear someone might say, "Well, button up your coat, you nut!"

I can hardly wait to be able to step out of the shower, wrap a towel around a relatively humanoid body, stand in front of the mirror, and feel rather cute while putting on my makeup. I'm jealous of the ease with which my husband wraps his towel around his waist. (Although, I must admit I enjoy looking at him in that particular outfit!) The largest towel I own (except a beach towel) won't wrap around me. No matter how I tuck and pull and squeeze, it won't reach. So I have to be careful when I shower. Since I can't stand the humiliation of Allen seeing me au naturel, I take my showers while he is gone or in bed. But who am I kidding? So I don't stand naked in front of him—he still has a pretty good idea that I'm "a little chubby."

I can hardly wait till I can sit in the driver's seat of the car after Allen has driven and not have to adjust the seat belt six-eight-ten inches larger. I always try to remember to readjust it back down to his size before I get out of the car. I absolutely hate for him to know how much fatter I am than he is. Again, who am I kidding?

I can hardly wait till the first person says, "Ohhhh—you've lost weight, haven't you?" I can hardly wait to be able to take a shower without having to lift rolls of fat to wash under. In fact, when I'm through with this diet, a shower will take me only half the time because I'll be only half the woman.

Wednesday, January 30, 1985
233 pounds

Today I finished reading *Anne of Green Gables*. The author made her so real, so alive, that I feel I have known Anne for years. What an inspirational book, what a delightful experience.

I had to write about the book because it was especially uplifting, with many important lessons. It made me feel lucky to be alive and healthy and able to do something about my future. Anne's feelings about life perfectly express my own feelings as I start out on this, my new life.

Each morning is glorious. It's almost frightening to think I may never have known this indescribable joy if I had never experienced such depths of depression and hell.

To change a habit, to overcome an addiction, to meet my own, personal Gethsemane face-to-face and win is incredibly uplifting. No one can understand unless he has gone through the fiery furnace. I've burned painfully for twelve years, suffering unspeakable torture. At last, I'm feeling the exquisite relief of leaping out of the furnace and jumping into the cooling, soothing pond of freedom. My joy couldn't be as intense if I hadn't burned for so long. The furnace has refined and hardened my resolve to stay in control.

Like Anne, I, too, have a destiny. I have a niche to fill and a role to play in this vast drama of human existence. I must become all that I can be. I'm going to pull myself up by my own bootstraps and succeed. I pray that somewhere down the road I can inspire even one person to do the same, to escape her own, self-imposed hell-jail. I suppose that could be the only feeling more elating than this experience of self-control.

Thursday, January 31, 1985
232 pounds

I've been giving a lot of thought to *why* fat people eat. I believe there are four main reasons: (1) habit, (2) hunger, (3) emotions, (4) irrational frenzy.

Habit. Probably the most insidious of all. You're not hungry, you don't necessarily like the food. You don't even realize what you're doing—but you continually shovel it in. Now, here's a lament for fat housewives everywhere: we can't get away from food. It is impossible! We housewives are responsible for buying, storing, cooking, and serving the wretched stuff. Not once a week, but *three times a day*! We are victims of our lot in life. As we clear breakfast dishes, we unconsciously clear all leftovers, all scraps, all spills—not into the garbage—but, gasp, into our mouths. As we make lunch for our little ones, without thinking about it, we pop a whole peanut-butter-and-jelly sandwich into our mouths, one tiny quarter at a time. As we clean up after lunch, we, again, simulate a human garbage can; before we put the lid on the peanut butter, we dip the knife in one more time. Ditto for the jam. "Oops, a few chips fell out of the bag," and "Why bother putting the last of the milk away?" Can you begin to see a little problem here? You ain't seen nothin' yet!

Preparing dinner is a regular feast. I'm not talking about eating dinner; I'm talking about *preparing* dinner. "Hmmmm, this gravy needs a little more salt." A few additional tastes and the gravy is perfect. I'm talking serving-spoon-size tastes. Then, when all is well with the gravy, a few more heavy-duty slurps prior to putting it on the table insure its edibility. Slice the cheese—eat two slices. Make a fruit salad—take several bites of each fruit you slice. Taste this, try that, here a little, there a little.

Now, for dessert. (Ohhhh, poor little children and hubby mustn't be deprived!) How about oatmeal cookies? I have *such* a recipe. And where do you think I obtained this dastardly combination of ingredients? From a fat friend, of course! (I should burn it!) Before the first cookie sheet comes out of the oven, I've eaten at least a dozen cookies—in the form of dough. Then I'll sample a few cookies before dinner to make sure they're done to perfection. Oh, how we deceive ourselves. Somehow, it's easy to snitch cookies. If you sit down and cut yourself a whole piece of cake, which necessitates getting out a plate and fork . . . now, that's *really* being a pig! But a cookie is so small, so convenient, so easy to rationalize. The average fat housewife easily downs two dozen before she serves them to her family.

But remember—and this is the important thing: we're talking *habit* here. Most of this nibbling is done without thinking, simply because the food is there. The pathetic part is when the out-of-control housewife then sits down with the family and *eats a full meal*. Habit nibbling is a serious problem. I, myself, and many other fat housewives I've talked to frequently eat all day long. Many days, not more than fifteen minutes go by without our popping something into our mouths. Like it or not, hungry or not, we pass by the drainboard, the food is there, we eat it.

Hunger. That is almost a joke. I've gone years without my stomach growling. Really now, how can you be hungry if you eat every fifteen minutes? No, hunger is not a significant problem for the fat person. It would humiliate me to say, "I'm hungry," let alone, "I'm starving." I assume everyone within earshot thinks, "It's about time, you little oinker. You could live a year on that lard you're carrying."

As I'm writing this today, I wonder . . . should I confess all? What I am about to disclose is mortifying. In my church, on the first Sunday of each month, we are asked to fast two meals and give the money we save to the poor. Fasting helps the needy and also helps cleanse our souls and draws us closer to God. It is mortifying to admit this, but I eat anyway. One little day a month, and I can't control my hideous appetite. Not even for two meals.

I pretend to fast, but I slip into the kitchen and snitch a bite of this or that. Anything I can cram and chew quickly. Then, I have to be sneaky about the smell of food on my breath. Fasting is good for me and I want to do it, so I feel miserable about cheating on myself.

How do you think I feel when I talk about fasting with my children? When I tell them to think of all the people who are hungry in the world each and every day? When I tell them a great big child like themselves can skip a couple of meals one Sunday a month without complaint? In reality, my children are unusually good about fasting without complaint. Their willing attitude adds to my guilt.

See what I mean? Fat people rarely eat out of real hunger. We never allow ourselves to get hungry. Not even on Fast Sunday!

Emotions. The main problem with emotional eating is that you can binge over *any* emotion. Many times when I was furious with Allen, I would storm into the kitchen, grab the first fattening thing I could find, and "show him a thing or two!" I'm afraid that at 263 pounds, all I "showed him" was fat.

I ate because I was frustrated with my children. Why wouldn't they clean their rooms? Why didn't they fold their clothes neatly? Why this? Why that? Why not eat? Several candy bars later, I'd call them all in and say, "Won't you please behave? Why do you think I'm so fat? I can't take all this pressure!" Can you believe that—from a mother? Blaming her poor, innocent children.

Humiliation has also caused me to pig out on numerous occasions. Many times I've caught a glimpse of some past acquaintance I haven't seen for ten years—no, haven't seen for 100 pounds. (We fat people measure time by our weight.) So why didn't I say hi to my old friend? Why? Because I'd rather die first! I am so humiliated, I pretend I never recognized them . . . then I go home and eat a dozen doughnuts.

Why would anyone eat as a reaction to the emotion of happiness or relief? When I've accomplished something big, when I'm finished with a critical project or program, I am compelled to grab a piece of cake, a root-beer float, anything to help celebrate.

I tell you, I will eat over *any* emotion! After having an especially wonderful, loving experience in bed with my husband, what do I sometimes do? Climb out of bed and go eat a candy bar! Gee whiz!

Eating as a reaction to an emotion is sheer stupidity! The fact that I have stopped doing just that is one reason I am currently feeling so marvelous. For over three weeks, I've controlled my own body. I've been acting instead of reacting.

Irrational frenzy. The normal person would call this a craving, but the truly obese know it's pure, unadulterated frenzy. Call it addiction, if you prefer. You're doing something, it could be anything at all—washing, dusting, reading, watching TV—and suddenly you're attacked by that ugly monster. Frenzy rears its cruel face at you and bites!

You run toward the kitchen like a person possessed. "Where's some chocolate? I must have chocolate. I'd trade my wedding ring for an M&M. I'd sell my soul for a Hershey's Kiss." You tear the food out of the cupboard where you keep the chocolate chips. Surely, there is at least one little chip that fell out of that last bag. You don't care how old or stale it is, as long as it's chocolate! None there. Absolute panic grips your throat! It's late. The stores are closed. You can hardly breathe. Surely, somewhere in the world there's an available piece of chocolate. You'd go anywhere, do anything, to find it. With one exception. You can't bring yourself to say "Please, God, please help me find some chocolate." But, oh! You come so close to saying it.

Then your eyes spot the mixer. Ah! Relief in sight. You can make some chocolate frosting! But can you make it soon enough? Will it be sufficiently whipped before your heart stops beating? You tear around the kitchen like a maniac for the ingredients. You measure as carefully as your trembling hands will allow. Before the beaters come to a complete stop, you have a bite in your mouth. Ah! Heaven. Slowly that chocolate sensation floods through your mouth, then down your throat. It flows to every little fat cell of your body. After half a cup, your heart rate is normal again. Your breathing becomes regulated. Your eyes are no longer popping out. Now you can settle down and *enjoy* another half cup of the pure, rich, sugary stuff, though you know you'll pay the price in the middle of the night. You'll be devilishly sick and swearing over and over that you will never, *ever* eat that kind of garbage again. Yes, folks, as you can see, that's no mild craving—that's irrational frenzy!

Why does frenzy strike without warning? Without regard to race, religion, sex, age, size, or anything else? I don't know. I keep hoping there is some dastardly deed from my childhood I am forgetting, and when I remember it, I will be cured of my bizarre cravings.

But in the meantime, I must remember this important diet principle: Before you put a single crumb into your mouth, decide which of the four reasons for eating is motivating you. Are you really hungry? If yes, fine, go ahead, as long as it's on your Daily Menu. Are you eating out of habit? That's one you can easily control by talking to yourself. There's a good chance that you are not especially fond of whatever you were about to pop into your mouth. Thinking for a second makes it possible to do without those calories! Are you eating because of an emotional crisis or because you feel you deserve a reward? Stop! Get a grip! Write a letter, sing a song, play the piano, or yell, but for heaven's sake, don't eat.

And what if you come to the realization that you are eating out of pure, irrational frenzy? Look out! You're in trouble. Talking to a friend or yourself doesn't always help. I've felt it twice in the past three weeks. It's preferable to satisfy the bizarre need, so be prepared. Have some baked chicken in the fridge (or something else you can really sink your teeth into), popcorn you can pop, diet pop already chilled—anything you love that's low-calorie and readily available. Both times frenzy struck, I snorted around till I ate something yummy, yet not off my diet.

Today I was proud because I'd taken the time to analyze why I was about to eat. And know what? I put the food down. I wasn't hungry, so I wasn't eating! Whenever something sounded or smelled good, I'd think to myself, "The less I eat, the more I lose."

September 30, 1991. My brother Stephen recently finished a preliminary review of my diary, prior to publication. His most important comment to me personally was this, "Gosh, Rose, I keep reading over and over how you go crazy on chocolate. I'm telling you now, you can never have chocolate again. I mean never. *You must believe me. It's a killer for you. As of today, I've been dry for twenty weeks. The next time you have a candy bar, call*

me, and I'll come over and have a six-pack with
you. It's that critical."

He is right. I have not had a bite of chocolate
since he first called me six days ago. I am seriously
trying to look at it in the same way an alcoholic
looks at alcohol. It is not on my menu anymore.
Never again. It is hard for me to fathom that. Never
again caressing an Almond Joy or a Baby Ruth.
Saying good-bye forever to Butterfingers and Kit
Kats. But I must. Chocolate is a drug to me. I have
an adverse reaction to it. Not only do I break out
in ugly fat, but my mind goes bonkers, and I eat
till I get sick. So all you chocolate bars out there,
fare-thee-well. No, Stephen, I shall never ask you
to drink with me. I love you too much! Thanks.

Saturday, February 2, 1985
230 pounds

It's been a glorious, marvelous day! I've lost twenty pounds
in less than three weeks! I've lost one-sixth of my total
"lardo," the fattest, greasiest sixth of all.

I had to see if one of my "smaller" dresses would fit me.
Maybe I could wear something different to church tomorrow.
It was sensational to slink into a dress I hadn't worn in over
a year. (Okay, I didn't exactly slink into it. Face it, dear
heart, at 230 pounds you can't slink into anything!)

Then I tried on everything—everything! You see, mine is
the perfect example of the typical fat person's closet. You
know—all the fat clothes I can barely squeeze into on one
end, with the rest I've outgrown taking up 90 percent of the
total space. The sad part is to think how many times I've
gone through my closet in the past and boxed up everything
that wouldn't fit. (What a depressing experience—talk about
self-hatred!) Then, somehow, it happens all over again. Grad-
ually, the clothes that take up the one little end—the clothes

I can barely squeeze into—become the 90 percent that no longer fit. The one little end now contains clothes a size or two larger than a few months ago. But I escaped that vicious cycle! I broke out.

It was awesome cleaning out my closet. It evoked feelings different from any I've ever known. It was different from my wedding day, when everything was white and perfect. It was different from giving birth to one of my precious babes, when the instant joy of motherhood overshadowed any previous pain. It was different from being selected a Rose Festival princess, when all cameras and eyes turned to me with admiration. Can I satisfactorily describe it? It was like lying on the beach as the waves come in. But instead of water, they were waves of joy and anticipation. First, the waves only tickled my toes, but they slowly climbed higher and higher. Then, finally, they were bursting over me, crashing down upon me, filling me with sheer delight.

I could hardly breathe. I had to dance and jump around. I had to run and look at myself in the mirror. I had to let out little screams of elation. What a different sensation from the last time I cleaned my closet and boxed up everything too *small*. How I cried then, how I hated myself! But no tears today, no depression. Only the stimulating anticipation of thinness!

Thursday, February 7, 1985
229 pounds

Wow!—pant—do I—pant—feel good! I just exercised for about ten minutes. I need to work up to thirty, but even ten minutes makes my heart rate rise till I tingle all over. I feel so exuberant right now, I'm amazed it's so difficult to start exercising each day.

It finally happened today, my first, unsolicited "You look like you've lost weight." "Oh, yes," I answered casually, as if I hadn't been waiting for this comment for a million years. "I've lost twenty-one pounds." Almost ho-hum. As if I didn't expect the heavens to open then and there, with angels breaking forth in a glorious "Hallelujah Chorus." I acted nonchalant, but inside I was shouting for joy, jumping up and down, patting myself on the back.

Finally, someone noticed! People will soon start watching closely to see if I'll keep on losing, or if I return to my old Miss Piggy self. I'll show them all. I don't think anyone believes I'll do it.

I can show people when I really want to. Take Allen, for instance. When we were first married, I was a size ten, five feet eight inches, about 140 pounds. But Allen used to complain that I was too fat, that I should go on a diet. He was one person I showed. Yup. I showed him what *fat* is! Believe me, after living with a 263-pound raving maniac for twelve years, he is going to think 140 pounds seems just fine; he might even call me skinny.

While I was exercising tonight, I started laughing out loud. Picture me, a mere 229 pounds, sitting on the floor in my exercise clothes, legs stretched out in front of me, trying to touch my nose to my knee. That mental picture alone is hilarious. The fat on my stomach makes it impossible to bend over very far, but the thing that made me laugh out loud was my inability to breathe when I tucked my head down. I kept being smothered by my own bosom. One does have to keep a sense of humor as a fat person. If you couldn't occasionally laugh at some of the problems fat causes in your life, you would continually be crying. I must say, it's a lot easier to laugh while on the way *down* the scale. If I were gaining at this time, nothing would be funny.

Saturday, February 9, 1985
229 pounds

There were a few moments last night when I felt like a fairy princess—like a real, bona fide Cinderella! It was divine.

Allen and I attended a dance at church, and I fell in love with a new man. He was a delightful partner, unspeakably handsome and perfectly groomed. Why, Allen would never dance like that!

But it *was* Allen! He whirled and twirled me around till I, at 229 pounds, felt almost light on my feet. There were a few moments when our steps were perfectly synchronized. It was a feeling I'd never before experienced. It was as if we were one person creating graceful, beautiful movements on the dance floor. Then my energetic partner proceeded to hit an all-time high while dancing to "New York, New York." He was electrifying! Was this the rather quiet, dignified man with whom I had come in? Why, he was Fred Astaire or Gene Kelly, but certainly not Allen Green.

I had a revelation right there on the dance floor, a revelation that would have left me in tears one month ago, before I was in control. Before I was on my way down. Why, after living with this man for almost fourteen years, there was another side to him that I did not know. He had more feeling and rhythm and zest for life than I had ever realized. And while I would have cried a month ago because I couldn't be part of it, last night I was thoroughly enthralled. I could visualize myself losing more weight and becoming part of that feeling and rhythm and zest. We would be able to share it and feel it together.

I was distressed and saddened by the inhibitions I had thrown over Allen because of my own self-consciousness and embarrassment over my weight. Thank goodness the fun of the evening overshadowed the shame and sadness I felt. I experienced euphoria as I contemplated shedding not simply 104 more pounds, but also the fears, frustrations, and life-sucking inhibitions those pounds have created! I have much to look forward to, many years to make up. I'm going to have superconcentrated good times. My life is going to become full to the brim. The more I lose, the more I'll gain. It was sensational last night, dancing with Allen, but it was only a tiny taste of the glory to come.

Wednesday, February 13, 1985
229 pounds

Why am I feeling so furious with myself right now? Several reasons:

1. I haven't lost any weight for twelve days. I've been so strict, I should have lost several pounds.
2. My husband has been sick in bed with the flu for four days. I love taking care of him and pampering him, but I lost my temper (I sure hope no one ever finds it!) and snapped out hurtful words. I'm sure I've made him feel guilty for being a burden; I hate myself for that.
3. I flew off the handle over my daughter's messy room. Now I hate myself even more. After all, she's only nine years old and has had a perfectly horrid example to follow all her life: me. So, I am overcome with yet more guilt, frustration, and self-hate. (Boy, that sounds like my cue to pig out.)
4. I'm mad that I have to baby-sit . . . and I'm mad that I'm mad. Baby-sitting is a fantastic way to earn money while staying home with my own children. I wouldn't trade the time I spend with my own babies for anything. It's watching someone else's children that is driving me nuts. Right now my sights are high for the future. The joys and delights of thinness loom before me like a giant beacon of light. It's hard being tied down to all these baby-sitting kids while I want to soar. While I want to write . . . and get my life organized.

I must concentrate on reasons to be thankful. I have many of those. I'm thankful my husband has not been diagnosed with a brain tumor, as in the case of my friend. I'm thankful none of my children are dwarfs, like those I saw on TV two nights ago. I'm thankful I'm enjoying a happy marriage to a loyal man instead of suffering through a miserable, ugly divorce.

I feel better now. It's amazing how I allow relatively insignificant matters to depress me. So there are a few clothes on the end of my daughter's bed—I should sweetly tell her to put them away. Why do I lose control in a moment, without any warning? Believe me, there's a lot more out of control in this fat girl's life than simply what goes into her mouth. In fact, what goes into my mouth has a lot to do with what comes out of it. Oh, to be escaping from that self-destructive cycle. I'm freeing myself from my negative, fat-induced behaviors. That will be as much of a joy as being thin.

Yesterday, one of my favorite day-care children, Marlie Wetzel, brought a bag full of chocolate hearts to share for a Valentine's treat! We're talking pure, rich, creamy chocolate here. Genuine chocolate, not chocolate-flavored. Chocolate that melts in your mouth and coats your throat and your senses with decadent delight—for maybe thirty seconds. Chocolate that then proceeds to coat your body with fat—blubbery, ripply, bouncy fat—and to coat your life with misery and hell. (Gee whiz! When I put it like that, it's no wonder I didn't eat any!)

Yet last year, the same little girl brought the same kind of chocolate hearts, and I—I'm so ashamed!—ate them all! All but one. I grudgingly divided it among the children. I had to. What would I do if Marlie's mother asked how the children liked the candy Marlie brought?

My usual method of feeding my habit was to hoard goodies, sharing very little. "What the kids don't know about, they can't ask for!" I'd say to myself. That beats the heck out of what some fat parents do. I swear, a certain kind of parent seems to get some comfort in encouraging her children to "eat that last cookie" or "have one more little piece of cake." Maybe she doesn't want to be the only fat person in the house. Maybe she's chagrined to be the only person stuffing her mouth with unnecessary, unhealthy calories. See that enormous lady over there with the pudgy little girl? What do you think she's feeding her daughter? Baked fish and carrot sticks?

Are you in a frame of mind to handle an ugly opinion? I

believe that parents who allow and often even encourage their children to overeat, or to eat highly fattening foods, are guilty of a most insidious form of child abuse. Think about it. The child who has been beaten or sexually abused has *some* moments of freedom. Not everyone knows of the hurt; few ever see the results. Occasionally, the child can enjoy herself and forget her personal trauma. But fat children? No relief, no hiding. *Everyone* knows. Daily ridicule. Being the last one picked for a team—*every* time. Losing *every* race. Wearing plain clothes. Every step reminding them that they are different because they waddle like ducks. Fat tummies keeping them from sitting comfortably close to their desks. Seeing the ugly reflection of fat cheeks in a mirror. On Valentine's Day, they live that song, "For those of us who knew the pain of Valentines that never came." Oh, my heart aches for all those Valentineless young people!

We all remember the fat kid in our classroom. Wasn't he teased unmercifully? Think back for a minute. I dare you to close your eyes and really think back. I bet you can remember his name. You can still visualize him or her, can't you? Wasn't it pathetic? Now, I ask you, is not this needless misery an insidious form of child abuse?

Please do not think for a minute that I put parents of overweight children in the same category with parents who beat or sexually abuse their children. But someone needs to speak up for these fat children. The result of *any* kind of child abuse is unfair cruelty, unnecessary human suffering. If for this reason alone, I must stick to my diet: to protect my children from my horrible example.

Smoking parents or drinking parents occasionally refrain from indulging in their ugly weakness. But fat parents are forever a sign of overindulgence, a perfect example of lack of self-control. Look around: fat adults usually raise fat children. My parents sure did! I am not going to do that. The fat cycle stops here, with me. I refuse to be the reason for anyone, especially my own children, to glutton out!

Saturday, February 16, 1985
230 pounds

I have achieved some spectacular successes this week. Wednesday night, while my sister Rebecca was at a wedding shower, I baby-sat her four-year-old daughter, Adriane. When Rebecca came to pick up Addie, she was carrying the prize she'd won at the shower, a homemade apple pie! "I'll leave half of it here," she said. "In fact, I'll taste it, and if it's not too good, I'll leave you the whole pie." Rebecca took a bite and declared it was "as good as Mom's"—and everyone knows my mother bakes the best apple pie ever! When Addie asked for a piece, Rebecca replied, "No, we'll each have a big piece when we get home. In fact (chuckle), there might not be any left when Daddy gets home tonight."

Only the truly obese could hear the tragic undertones in that sentence. My heart ached for Rebecca. But, at the same time, it sang with joy for me—because I have freed myself from her kind of jail. I knew I wouldn't take one taste of that apple pie, even if it were as good as Mom's. I generously shared it with the rest of my family. All five of them had a nice, normal-size piece. In the past, I would have kept that calorie-packed secret to myself. The pie would have been hidden, eaten, and all evidence disposed of deftly and expertly! I was proud of myself that night!

I am still such an obese humanoid, but I've grabbed on to the rope, and I'm slowly pulling myself out. Each pound I lose makes it that much easier to pull myself a little farther out of the mire. I feel optimistic. No more "fat jokes" while I eat goodies. No more pretending it's funny as I swallow brownies or fudge.

Only last Christmas, I sat with another fat lady at a party, and we devoured a disgusting amount of goodies. All the while, poor Allen sat by my side, watching. I hated myself anew each second. I detested every delicious, hideous morsel. I knew my poor husband must have been humiliated and disgusted, but . . . I kept eating. I tried to convince myself it was nibbling. Somehow, "nibbling" is okay. Surely, no one gets fat from nibbling. And, oh, how I clowned around with my fat friend. I feel embarrassed for myself even now, two months later. Never again; it's too terrible. Allen commented later that night that I seemed to "use" the fact that another fat person was eating goodies as an excuse to eat some myself. I knew he was right, but I hated him for making the comment.

Yesterday I put a desk in my bedroom. It's going to be *mine*. I'm thirty-two years old and never had a desk or special place of my own. I want to write down all my feelings. I want to pour out my heart and soul. I want to be motivated to stick to my diet. I want to remember the happy days, the thin days. I want to never, ever again hate myself, my life, everyone I see, the whole world even, just because I'm fat.

Sunday, February 17, 1985
227½ pounds

Oh, wow! I feel as if I've broken the sound barrier. I weigh 227½ today. That's the lowest I've weighed this time around. I'm through teeter-tottering and am on my way down again. There are many things I want to do, wear, and feel. You cannot imagine how exasperated I am with myself because I have eaten until my hands have become so fat that I can't wear my own wedding rings. I can't even get them past my first knuckle! Like the old gray mare, I ain't what I used to be. Every time I look at my rings, it's depressing to think of how worthless they are to me. To be able to slip them on my finger once again will be worth every sweet thing I've refused! Then, there's the pearl necklace Allen gave me for a wedding gift, the one that used to hang loosely around my neck. Ha! It chokes me now!

Yesterday, at the store, I tried on three hats. They were beautiful! Something inside me aches to wear pretty hats again, even though it's a "fat" no-no! But with my recent weight loss, I feel so much better, I ventured forth to the hat rack. I noticed a young lady standing a few feet away, kind of smirking at me. I could tell she was laughing at me, thinking I was a big, *fat* joke! Well, I'll show her! I *will* wear hats again—and look cute in 'em, too!

Let's face it, fat people shouldn't call attention to themselves in their dress or behavior. Our voluminous proportions are conspicuous enough. No hats—heaven forbid, people might stare more than usual. Faddish clothes designed for size-five models are definitely out for us. Anyone over a size twelve should lose the hot-pink anklets! And it should be illegal to sell gum to anyone overweight. The sight of those big, fat cheeks in constant motion turns the stomach of anyone with any class!

Tuesday, February 19, 1985
224 pounds

I love the scene from *Peter Pan* where Peter, Wendy, Michael, and John are all elevated—literally and emotionally. Literally, they are flying. Emotionally, they are also soaring. By that act of flying, they are feeling free of their cares and woes. And I'm right there with them. I'm flying. I have only ninety-nine more pounds to lose.

I can't think of anything but my new life before me. Today, I had a vivid picture come into my mind. I could see a baby being born. A baby who didn't know anything. A baby who was going through much pain and discomfort and didn't know of the opportunities and delights, the challenges and rewards to follow. A baby who didn't know about rainbows, or the first daffodils of spring, or summer showers, or mountains, or little streams, or first loves, or true loves, or Ferris wheels, or ocean waves, or anything.

Then here was I, thirty-two years old, seeing myself as a baby coming into this world. Only I already knew of all those things, and of myriads more. Of love and hate. Happiness and despair. Spiritual fulfillment and emptiness of the soul. I had experienced most every emotion imaginable. Here was I, in the birth canal again, already possessing the wisdom of those thirty-two years of trial and error. Ready to be born again. Oh, how many get a second chance? How many can detect—let alone kill—their Goliath? I'm so lucky. I'm so thankful. For a long time, I've been in a black tunnel with only a little light at the end. A tunnel I constructed torturously, pound by pound, with the very fat that encloses my body and puts my soul into continuous misery and hopelessness.

My vision has broadened from that little flicker of light, that tiny drop of hope in an immense ocean of fear, discouragement, and failure. Now I look out at an ocean full of joy, hope, elation. Wave after wave of pleasurable new life flows over me. The more I lose, the farther I come out of that dark, narrow tunnel.

As I write in my diary, I feel myself being filled with thoughts that are more than mine. Perhaps I can be an answer to another's prayer for help. I hope so. I hope my experience will be the beacon light for others who are suffering from this dread disease, this blight, this life-sucking monster.

My whole attitude has changed in the last five weeks. I *am* somebody. I *am* important. I *am* loved. I *do* have qualities and talents unique to me. The world is at my feet. I simply have to take the first step.

I love to write. As I do, I find bits and pieces of me expressing themselves, bits and pieces I didn't know before. It's fascinating. I like me. With each hour that I resist fattening things, I like me better . . . and the looks of me, too.

A funny thing happens whenever I discuss my weight with Allen. I subconsciously refer to my weight as if I were in the one-hundreds. I'll mistakenly say, "Oh, Allen, I weigh only 144-133-124 pounds this morning." Dear, sweet Al will always remind me, "You mean 244 or 233 or 224." Somehow, though it's been twelve years, my mind won't, can't, refuses to say any number in the two-hundreds. How dreadful it sounds. I *am* a skinny person trapped inside a fat body.

Today I sat in my car and buckled the seat belt. Can you imagine my delight when the tiniest adjustment allowed me to fasten it? Allen had driven the car last. He'd tightened the seat belt to *his* size. And, wow! It almost fit *me*. Now, I'm not saying it wasn't snug. (Okay, it was tight!) But with only a half-inch adjustment, it closed.

Wednesday, February 20, 1985
224 pounds

I get frustrated, even mad, when I think of the plight of the fat person. The horrible, disgusting, everyday plight: We are fat. We cannot get away from it. No matter where we go or what we do, even if we change our identity, we cannot escape it.

The thief, the drug dealer, even the murderer can turn a corner and be safe, be hidden. No one knows his crime. He could look like Joe Cool or Mr. Businessman. He can walk into a store, theater, business, church, or home, and no one knows. He can *hide* his guilt. But the fat person? Where can he go? What can he do? Everyone knows! And his sin? He simply eats too much! Somehow, it seems a bit of a severe punishment. The drug addict can get help and at least *look* normal in a short time. But me? If I moved to Australia and changed my name, I'd still be fat ol' me.

I experience the joy of release each time I slip on a pair of pants that were too tight a month ago, or when I put on a blouse that has obviously become too big since the last time I wore it, or when I'm walking and suddenly realize my legs don't rub together in the way they used to. Then I experience an elation that seems to lift me off the ground.

Yesterday, while grocery shopping with Allen, he suddenly made the comment, "Hey! You look better from behind.

Your coat doesn't balloon out like it used to.'' I decided to take that as a compliment.

Have you ever noticed how fat people often seem to be cold and are bundled up, even when no one else is? We fool ourselves by thinking that somehow we're not as fat with our coats on. No one can see our real shape. Ha! Ha! A tent is a tent is a tent! All the caftans, muumuus, shawls, and coats in the world can never hide what we are: fat! Out of control and dangerously obese. But if we couldn't fool ourselves occasionally, we'd all go crazy (as if we weren't that way most of the time, anyway!).

I can button my coat comfortably now. I find immense joy in that simple pleasure. When I clasp my hands, I'm amazed at how I can interlock my fingers closer together. I find myself clasping and unclasping my hands all day because my fingers feel almost bony.

Sunday, February 24, 1985
221 pounds

Two months ago, I thought I knew all there was to know about my husband of thirteen and a half years. I knew his moods, his likes, his loves, his temper, his gentleness—I thought I knew his everything. But this new, this thinner, in-control me is bringing out a new him.

When he looks at me, there is an intensity of love and adoration that has never been there before. Is he feeling from me the strength I feel when I'm in control? Is this new me so different from the old one, the depressed, out-of-control, frustrated humanoid, that he recognizes the inner strength it took for me to reach inside and pull myself together? Is it that strength and conviction he admires? He's never looked at me this way before.

Eureka! I suddenly realized how to describe it. The look I see on Allen's face is the look *I feel* as I look at him. I'm so in awe of him and his talents, abilities, and, most of all, his goodness. Could he possibly feel that way about *me*? Oh, dream come true! It seems impossible, but I see it in his eyes.

One day last week, he hugged me and exclaimed, "Oh, honey, I can put my arms around you and really hug you again. You're just a wisp!" Now, we all know that 220-ish pounds could never be wispy, but the thought delighted me. This twenty-pound loss has made a big difference. The next time you hug your sweetie, try putting a twenty-pound bag of flour between the two of you and see how close you can get. Not very sexy, is it?

And in the bedroom? Yes, there's a difference. Yes, the loving *is* better. How could it not be? Oh, fat people! Stop kidding yourself; you don't suffer alone! Your mate agonizes with you.

Saturday, March 2, 1985
221 pounds

I've been feeling down the last few days and it's time to do something about that. Thank goodness I haven't gone off my diet. This recent, depressed feeling has been a shrieking signal to my brain to sniff out chocolate, to dig up something sweet, to go for some poundage . . . but I haven't done it! I've kept control of my eating, if not my temper and emotions.

Tuesday, March 5, 1985
220 pounds

THE REASONS I WANT TO BE THIN

1. *For me!* I want to be able to skate, swim, dance, run, bike, participate in sports and—oh, who am I kidding? I want to be able to walk up one flight of stairs in my own house without breathing so hard I nearly hyperventilate! I want to show everybody that I *can* do it! I want to go to school,

church, and family reunions with my head held high. I want to wear hats and pretty clothes and feel good. I want to stop pretending that I don't recognize people I haven't seen for years . . . and stop praying that they don't recognize me. I want to stop making "fat-people" jokes intended to let people know that *I* know I'm fat. I want to start *living* again.

2. *For Allen!* I want him to be proud of me again. Years ago, when Allen introduced me as his fiancée to one of his old college friends, his friend kept exclaiming, "Allen, how did you ever get someone so *beautiful* to marry you?" Oh, how Allen beamed! I want him to beam again. I know he loves me. I know that he desires me emotionally. But I want—yes, I *need*—to be physically desired, even craved. I want to be the girl he married, not twice the girl. I want Allen, once again, to be able to do some of the things he used to enjoy— skiing, dancing, snorkeling—and to enjoy them with *me*.

3. *For my children!* I don't want them to be embarrassed of me. I don't want them to suffer the sometimes cruel remarks their friends may make. I have one haunting memory from the fourth grade. Susie Franklin was a girl in my class. She was overweight and rather unkempt. One day, there came to our classroom door a woman who was also overweight and not very well dressed. How it stung when a classmate said, "That must be Susie's mom." But, no, it was not Susie's mother. It was *my* mother. I wanted to crawl under my desk and never come out. My poor, little, nine-year-old spirit was experiencing two distinct emotions: humiliation and self-hatred.

I had reason to be humiliated. She *was* fat. She *was* poorly dressed. She wore no nylons. Her hair was frumpy, anything but stylish. I also had reason for hating myself. I couldn't bring myself to say, "No, that's *my* mom." I was relieved when they thought it *was* Susie's mother. I cried over that later, feeling terribly disloyal and sneaky. The memory still bothers me. I can't help wondering what my children are thinking when I visit their school. I want to spare them that kind of distress and the sad, enduring memories it brings.

I want to be able to play with my children. A few weeks

ago, I was talking to my little Matthew. He's seven. I told him that this summer I'd play tennis and ride bikes and do all sorts of fun things with him. He opened his eyes wide and gasped, "You mean, we'll even hike up Rocky Butte, and I can show you my fort?" His fort! I wanted to cry. He had never experienced a mother who could jump, climb, or hike. Oh, how could I deny my children and myself so much? I'd never seen my darling seven-year-old's little hideout. I can diet. I *will* do it. I mustn't wait until Matthew's grown up and it's too late for him to show me his fort.

4. *For other fat people!* Everyone has gifts and talents. Mine is the ability to give a speech that holds an audience in the palm of my hand. I can electrify people with my enthusiasm. I can motivate people to activity! And I am certain that in learning to conquer this dread disease of obesity, this monstrous madness, I can help others do the same. I can inspire those who have almost given up. I can use these past twelve hell years to good purpose.

I know firsthand what it's like! I have been there! There *is* a way back. There *is* hope for a real life. For fat people (I'm talking porkers here) life is a sit-on-the-bench observation of others having fun . . . like the butterfly that never escapes its cocoon, like the roll of film that never gets developed.

5. *For young people!* Who can young people look up to these days? Who can they emulate? Who can they imitate? Take a serious look at the movie stars, rock stars, TV idols. Really think for a second. Think of the vulgar and sick lyrics to many of today's most popular songs. Think of the evil, the pornography, the filthy words in nearly every movie. Yet these people are those in the limelight, those our children idolize.

I have a burning desire to do something distinguished. To fight and win a major war. To do something worthy of public notice. To be somebody. Young people need *someone* in the limelight to look up to who stands for right, for decency, for modesty, for motherhood and the American way! It's hard for any people, let alone young people, to look up to someone that they can barely look around. For them, too, I diet.

6. *For credibility with adults!* I have been an avid fighter of pornography for five years. I have been appalled by the dress standards—or lack of standards—of our schools, our television shows and commercials, and of our nation as a whole. But what impact can a blimp weighing over 250 pounds have on the subject of modesty? I mean, really. Can you imagine me rolling and bouncing up to a bikini-clad, 110-pound sex goddess and persuading her to cover up? Who would believe I'm anything but jealous? There are many issues with which I want to get involved, where I want my voice to be heard. But I'm so obviously out of control in my own life, what could my distorted opinion possibly be worth? "Who cares what that fat old biddy says?" But I do have some fine, even noble ideas—and I am yet going to have my day in court!

> *February 3, 1992. At the time I wrote the above entry, improving my health didn't seem an important reason for losing weight. I was only thirty-two years old. I thought I would be forever young. But as the big 4-0 looms hideously before me, I realize I am headed on a crash course with middle age. And yes, losing weight for health reasons has become extremely important to me. In fact, only last month, a forty-six-year-old friend of mine had a stroke. I am sure it was more than coincidence that this friend was extremely obese.*

Wednesday, March 6, 1985
220 pounds

When I was exceedingly fat, I had only one dress that fit. I made sure it was clean on Saturday, and then I knew I had something to wear for Sunday. Yesterday, while getting ready for church, I had five different dresses to choose from! I couldn't decide what to wear. It has been a long, depressing time since I've experienced that "girlish" decision.

It was horrible when I had only one decent pair of pants to my name. The other ones were all worn out—guess where? They were worn out between my legs. It's disgusting for me to mention it at all, but the inside top of each pant leg was totally worn out. There was a hole about two inches in diameter on either side. Those two big holes were created because my legs were so fat that they rubbed together every step I took and wore the fabric out. Yup, that's what I've done—worn holes in my pants! It just makes me sick.

Saturday, March 9, 1985
220 pounds

I talked with Allen for almost two hours this morning. It's interesting that I find myself telling him things about myself that I'd never consciously realized. It fascinates me that the more I lose, the more I can reveal "fat secrets" to him. Things I would have died mentioning before this weight loss are now fun and exciting to share with him. I've noticed another significant phenomenon: Because I'm on my way down, I can do things that would otherwise embarrass me. If I were at this exact weight, but on my way *up*, I wouldn't want to talk to Allen about losing weight. I would never, never have tried on a hat in a store. It's crazy; I'm ninety-three pounds overweight, but I almost feel cute and little.

When I'm in the driver's seat of a car and have to lean across to open the door, I can do it! If that seems crazy to mention, then you've never been fat. You don't know—and I'm glad you don't—how one has to squirm, shift, grunt, stretch, and inevitably rip the seams out under the arms, trying to reach across the car. It sends a little thrill of accomplishment through me as I now easily lean over and lift the lock. I don't have to concentrate on how to move most easily, and I never hear threads snapping anymore.

As I sat in the car yesterday, I was suddenly aware that my coat was roomy around the shoulders. No more tightness up under my arms; no more cutting off the circulation to my hands. I felt my shoulders move inside my coat. I'd forgotten how that feels.

I told Allen how I sit in our women's meeting at church each Sunday and count all the fat ladies, from one end of the room to the other. I don't know why I do. I don't think I have ever given it a second thought. Until this morning. Why *do* I count the fat ladies? I must find a sense of comfort in it. I'm not glad that any certain person is fat. I'm devastated for her. But I do find refuge in the fact that I am only one of so many fat people in the room. It helps me to endure the shame, the total humiliation of sitting there with my stomach in my lap. If I fold my arms in front of me, I look like an armored tank, but it's uncomfortable to let them hang. I can't clasp my hands in my lap, because there's no lap left after my stomach spills over.

How do I keep my knees together in a ladylike fashion? You try putting two cans of shortening between your upper legs and see how hard it is! With the ham hocks I'm wearing, it's about as easy for me to cross my legs as it is for a full-grown pig to do so. Think about it. When a woman's thighs reach a certain dimension, it's physically impossible for her to lift one leg over the other. It won't reach. It's an unpleasant thought. It's a more unpleasant feeling.

However, before you reach that disgustingly fat point, it's possible to kind of push one leg over the other, using your hands. But you need to be aware of two things when doing so: (1) your leg is so heavy that the pressure of all that weight will cut off the circulation in both legs within a few minutes; (2) you must hold the top leg in place with your hand or—like a tight spring—your leg will "poing" off, out of control, and possibly kick someone sitting in front of you.

Then there's the act of sitting itself. Let's assume the chair has armrests (that takes care of where to put my fat arms) and I'm wearing pants (that takes care of the need to keep my knees together). How can I hide the four inches of pure,

pure, unadulterated fat hanging over the chair on both sides? Or the puffy derriere that pokes through between the seat and the backrest? Or the hips that bulge out between the seat and the armrests?

What we have here is self-inflicted torture—trying to tuck in my stomach, keep my knees together, and somehow keep my backside from poking out through the various chair openings. I can feel the stupid, senseless suffering even now. I am again reminded of Dickens' *A Christmas Carol*. All the ghosts moaning miserably, wrapped about by chains forged with their own hands. We obese are inwardly moaning miserably—wrapped about by fat forged with our own "hands to mouths."

Now, as my body changes, so does my outlook. I'm not sitting there depressed anymore. Oh, I'm not kidding myself. I'm still extremely obese, but I won't be for long. Yes, I still count the fat ladies. But now, I'm alive and anxious for the future, waiting for my tiny bud of life to open and reveal the beautiful rose within. The me. The me that I want to be—that I *will* be.

> *July 8, 1991. My sister Debbie recently read this entry. "Rosemary!" she exclaimed, "I count all the fat ladies, too. I can't believe it. I sit there and mentally go down each row and make note of the fatties." So now I know that I've been counted by at least one person. Well, in three months, I'd like to see anyone count me fat.*

Night before last, I attended a PTA meeting. I now hold my head higher and smile more. That in itself is wondrous. But it was the proverbial frosting on the cake when the joyous flood of realization hit me: "I'm not the fattest person in the room!" Now, I wouldn't wish this dread curse on anyone. But if there is a person in the neighborhood who is already fat, I'm thankful she attended this particular meeting. And there were at least three ladies at that meeting who were fatter than I am! I was happy, thankful I'd been able to drop thirty-two of my little tormentors. It spurred me on to want to lose more!

Last night I experienced something I knew was inevitable. I'm sure all the fat people who know me will be happy for me to lose weight. But I also know that they will hate me for it. You see someone who has been fat forever suddenly break the bonds, spring the lock, so to speak. When you first notice it, you're sure it's your imagination. But week after week, this old fat friend, or acquaintance, melts before your eyes. And you hate her. You're jealous. You're angry. She has been fat for so long, if she can do it, my goodness, anyone can. So why don't you? You *can't* ask her how she did it; you won't even bring it up. You just avoid looking her in the eyes anymore, and you consider her an enemy of sorts; she has obviously defected to the other side.

I had that experience with someone last night. That "someone" was Melissa, a friend who lives up the street. She's also very obese. Two months ago, we laughed, joked, and disgusted ourselves over our own fat. I waited to tell her about my diet until after I'd lost fifteen pounds. I remember telling her, "You know, after I lose fifty pounds, I'll look better than you. Better get on the ball."

"Oh, yes," she laughed. We both knew it would infuriate her if that happened. Now that I've lost thirty-two pounds, I *do* look better than she does. And it's no longer funny. It isn't going to happen, it *has* happened. When I told her last night that I'd lost thirty-two pounds, she wrinkled up her nose and said, "I hate you." I knew what she meant. She didn't actually hate me. She hated my ability to lose weight, and she hated herself for not doing it. She hated life, work, men. Oh, yes, I knew what she meant. But it was a sad moment for me, because I realized I could no longer talk about weight with her. I could never again tell her how much I'd lost or how fantastic I felt. I had to face the fact that my weight loss also resulted in a loss of part of my relationship with Melissa. I'd obey one of my own "rules for thin people" and never bring up weight with this fatter-than-me person again.

Sunday, March 10, 1985, 10:00 A.M.
219 pounds

Occasionally, we all find ourselves at the edge of the cliff of control. One more step and there will be nothing beneath our feet. We will lose control and go berserk. But the decision to take that last step is ours, and we are ultimately responsible for our out-of-control actions.

Well, yesterday I was out-of-control angry with Allen. Whoever coined the phrase "hell-cat" must have known someone like me. I am not exactly Mary Poppins when I'm angry. I could feel the fires raging inside me. Allen had mocked my diary. While he was outside washing the car, he yelled out for all the world to hear that not only was I fat, I was also mean, and why didn't I go write about *that* in my diary. Oh, talk about Mount St. Helens. I would show him.

I marched into the house. "Mock my diary would you? Ohhhh! You went too far that time, buster!" I flounced into my bedroom, removed the pages from my diary, marched back down the hallway, grabbed some matches, turned on the gas starter in the fireplace, and proceeded to burn page after page. I watched each paper burn. Oh, I was so clever. I felt so smug. Allen would be infuriated. But most of all, I showed him. He would be sorry. He would stop making fun of me and my writing.

As the papers turned black and became ashes, I felt a marvelous sense of victory. I'd won the battle. As each page burst into flames, the heat it generated was richly rewarding. As I watched them burn, I realized there was part of me on each page of my diary. Hours of my life. Pieces of my personality. Glimpses of my soul. My dreams for the future.

But none of that mattered at the time, just as long as I could hurt Allen. Maybe I could even make him realize how much he'd wounded me! Ah! Done in the nick of time. Allen came into the kitchen. He didn't know yet. He commented on the fire. (Such an unsuspecting lamb.) Then, as I abruptly left the kitchen, he almost choked with realization. He gasped out one word at a time as he asked, "What . . . did . . . you . . . burn?" I didn't answer. I was reveling in my revenge. He asked Tiffany, "What did she burn?"

I heard Tiffany reply, "Some papers with writing on them." Ah! Sweet, sweet revenge.

Allen rushed down the hallway, his voice raspy with fear. "Did you burn your diary?"

And now for the coup de grâce: "It was *my* diary—I could do what I wanted with it!" There! At last he knew. "You're never going to make fun of it again." I turned and saw a look of agony on his face that I'd never seen before. Truly. His reaction was a knife plunging through me. I *had* hurt him, but not as I expected. He didn't get mad and lose his temper.

His face crumpled as he cried, "Oh, you fool. What have you done? I feel such a sense of loss. The world has lost something incredible, something it desperately needed."

I was shocked. My plan had backfired. I did not expect this. I thought he would be angry because of the loss of something of potential monetary value. But he showed concern for *my* words. For the me I'd been able to put on paper. He had actually said, "The world has lost something incredible. . . ." Was he seriously talking about anything *I* could write? What a compliment.

At that moment, I was thrilled . . . and thankful. Thrilled, for I knew Allen meant it. Thankful, for I had burned only newspapers! If you were fooled, it was because I left out one tiny detail: I did take the pages out of my notebook, but I hid them and grabbed some old newspapers instead. I'd never acted out something like that before, but it was an incredible experience. As I sat before the fire, putting in page after page of newspaper, I realized how important my diary is to me. It matters not what comes of it later. To me it is priceless. To me . . . it *is* me!

It was a climactic moment when I told Allen I'd only burned newspapers! What an actress! What a scene. Jane Fonda, eat your heart out. Imagine, me in a starring role. I must admit, I loved it. I ate it up. I'd fooled everyone. ("I want to thank you for this Oscar. I worked extremely hard for it!'')

The relief on Allen's face was as unfeigned as the torture had been. But he had to know for sure. "Where is it?"

"I hid it. I wanted to make you feel how hurt I was by what you said."

"It worked. I was sick."

Curtain closes on couple as they talk over their ridiculous argument. Book closes on this entry.

Sunday, March 10, 1985, 10:30 P.M.
219 pounds

Yesterday, while I was talking with my cousin, she asked, "Haven't you just lost some weight?" Because it's the main thing on my mind these days (I'd rather have fat on my mind than on my body!), I was delighted that she brought up the subject. My cousin was excited for me. I know she was. But during our conversation, she made one of the unbelievably inane statements that are often made by friends of dieters.

Okay. Here's a fat person. Probably been fat for years. This rotund person finally decides to do something about it. She starts dieting. She loses some weight, twenty or thirty pounds. Maybe half or a quarter of what she needs to lose. Of course, dieting comes up in the conversations of this little chub-o-lard. And, of course, her friends ask the inevitable, "What weight do you want to get down to?" The faithful dieter replies, "X pounds." Then comes the all-time discouraging, unmotivating, thoughtless response from the alleged friend: "Oh, no, you mustn't lose that much weight. You'd be too thin!"

Oh, *please*! Give me a break. We are talking twelve years of fat and 140 extra pounds of beef on the hoof here. Do you think I would mind if someone thought me too thin? Do you think I'd feel insulted if an anonymous caller told me to eat a few Butterfingers between meals? Do you think I would write a new book on the despairs of being a size seven? "You mustn't lose that much weight," my eye!

Let's be realistic for a minute. How many people do you know who have ever been 100 pounds overweight and then dieted till they looked vaguely normal, let alone thin? Or too thin? Can you honestly name one? I can't! So what are the odds of my ever making it? Lousy. What are the odds of my losing even another thirty pounds? Lousy!

So, for heaven's sake, why discourage the poor fatty before she quits of her own accord and goes blimping back up the scale? If I say I'm going to reach 125 pounds, respond with, "Wow! That's great." Help me. Believe in me! Don't add one single, negative note. If I am too thin at 125, don't worry or fret; I'll be the one who has to cry myself to sleep every night (in my sexy, new, black negligee).

Tuesday, March 12, 1985, 5:23 P.M.
220 pounds

I am so upset, I'm trembling. I am totally unable to comprehend the conversation I just had. It all started a few weeks ago, when I called for an appointment with Kaiser Permanente, my health-care provider. I wanted to see a dietitian. I felt it wise, as I planned to lose 125 pounds. I had a few serious concerns about the need to be taking vitamins while dieting. Mind you, two months ago, I could never have made the call. As a fat person, I have to muster up astounding courage to finally ask a doctor for help. It's easy to try appetite suppressants, crazy fad diets, or mail-order, instant weight-loss gimmicks. No honest commitment necessary. But a doctor, an honest to goodness "you-are-too-fat-here-is-a-diet-now-stick-to-it" doctor, that's serious business. Making that phone call is positively mind-boggling. You even hang up a couple of times before dialing the complete number.

Holding my breath, my heart pounding, trying to use my very thinnest voice, I asked for an appointment with a dietitian. The receptionist said I had to get a referral from a doctor before I could see a dietitian. Oh, tragedy! Think of it: a desperate fat person calling for help, suffering from the humiliation of having to say, "Here I am, Mrs. Blimpo herself. Show me how to eat like a normal human being. Please help me lose weight and be a real, true person again—or I will kill myself."

And the response? There was a twang in her voice like that of a recording: "You'll have to get a physical exam first and be referred to the dietitian by a doctor." Oh, get real! I'm 125 pounds overweight. It doesn't take a doctor to discover it! Any four-year-old could tell me I need to go on a diet!

"But you must have your blood pressure checked, you must have your cholesterol level counted, you must . . . you must . . . you must." If I hadn't been faithful on my diet and already lost some weight, I'd have hung up the phone and found a sharp razor blade. Naaah, I'd have probably whipped up a double batch of chocolate frosting!

Doctors, of all people, should want to help the obese. Doesn't anyone in the whole Kaiser Permanente organization realize that a fat person is one of the most desperate people on earth? The slightest problem will trigger an eating binge like a match ignites gasoline. These so-called professionals! Don't they know anything about real people? That "see a doctor" line is all a fatty needs to hear. "See a doctor" is a simple sentence to normal people. But to the obese? Think about it. It *really* says: Take off all your clothes. Put on this ridiculous little apron affair that barely comes around your hips, let alone your backside. Remain in this seminaked state till the doctor comes in and gives you an exam. He'll have to lift several rolls of blubber trying to find the real you. If he says turn over, or scoot down, you'll feel like a quivering bowl of Jell-O, with no muscles or control, as you try hefting your massive body. Then he'll push, prod, do a "tsk-tsk" with his tongue, and finally eject his "You really need to lose some weight."

I've had nurses give me some painful shots before, but not one hurt me like the time a nurse told me, "Honey, you're too pretty to be so heavy.'' Does she honestly feel she paid me a compliment? I hated her.

"Yeah, well you're too crude to be a nurse!'' I didn't say it, but I wish I had.

Or how about the doctor examining me for headaches. I can see him clearly even now, with his fingers laced behind his head, leaning back in his chair. "You are much too heavy. Why don't you go on a diet?'' Oh! Hate, hate, hate. It had nothing to do with my headaches. How dare he? And so cold, so mean—"Why don't you go on a diet?''

I started to get tears in my eyes as I responded, "It's just so difficult—'' Then he might as well have hit me over the head with a stethoscope when he interrupted with, "Well, it's not our concern here, anyway.'' Nice guy. Who brought it up in the first place?

The point is, the Kaiser receptionist made it seem impossible to see a dietitian, so I hung up. It's significant to remember that had this been a few weeks ago, I would have rushed to the store as fast as I legally could. I would have grabbed my favorite six. I would have hurried home. I would have locked my bedroom door and crashed onto my bed. I would have opened a good book. I would have chomped down on the goods! And I would have been justified because nobody cared, not Allen, not the doctors. It was their fault. I had tried. What else was there to eat in the house?

Oh, the beaten path to my bed! How many times the aforementioned justification had taken place! But this time? No way! This time was different. I'm in control. I hold the keys and the answers.

So, I called the Kaiser customer-service office and complained. I described the situation to the lady who answered. She was sorry. She'd see if she could get the dietitian to call me. I wouldn't leave my name and number. The whole experience was too mortifying. When I called her back, she informed me I could call the dietitian myself. I did. "She's not available; could you please leave your name and number?'' Oh, brother. I took a deep breath and thought for a second. If I hung up right now, no one would ever know who I was. But I did want some answers. Okay, I left my name. I bet they've written all over my file, *Beware this wacko fat lady!*

Ten long days later, the dietitian returned my call. She answered a couple of questions, but boy-oh-boy, was she a hard case. Did she ever have a chip on her shoulder.

"You need to see a doctor. You need to drink more water." (No acknowledgment of the two quarts I drink each day.) "The exercises you do are of no worth. You are losing weight too fast. You need to come to one of my diet meetings." (With 200 other fat, out-of-control humans? No thanks!) "You will gain all of your weight back. You should definitely not diet until a doctor has checked your blood pressure, taken your temperature, given you a menu."

Don't dietitians ever have heart-to-heart talks with any of their obese patients? Don't they realize I'm out of breath just walking from my bedroom to the bathroom? Don't they know I have constant back pain and body aches? Don't they know that after I sit down on the floor for a few minutes, the circulation in one or both of my legs is completely cut off and I can hardly move for five minutes? Don't they consider the careful calculations I must make to simply bend over and pick up something off the floor? Don't they have any idea that I sound like an elephant walking down the hallway in the morning, before my grotesque body limbers up? Don't they know I only *dream* of exercising; I never really *do* it? Don't they know that sometimes I stuff the fattening food in my mouth so fast that I can't even taste it and literally choke on it in my hurry to hide the evidence?

Do they honestly mean that eliminating chocolate, ice cream, and potato chips from my diet is dangerous? It seems that when doctors hang their degrees on the wall, it somehow gives them the license to hang all fat people out to dry! I have not yet met one doctor who is wise, empathetic, or realistic about obesity!

The dietitian said that one problem with dieting without a doctor's supervision is that the dieter almost always gains it back. Well, open your eyes, bozo. Think about it. Doctor, schmoctor! The only reason anyone gains back any significant amount of weight after dieting is because the person eats like a crazy fool again.

Dietitian: "That's probably often the case, but some people can't eat as much as other people without gaining weight." Oh, please! Spare me the thyroid routine. Of *course* no two people can eat the exact same thing with the exact same results. But get real! If an obese person says all he eats is one egg for breakfast, a green salad for lunch, and two pieces of chicken for dinner, and still gains weight . . . he's lying. It's that simple. Maybe he can fool a doctor who has only ten years of medical training, but he can't fool me. I've been to the depths of hell for my education, for these scars—and burned there for twelve years!

Needless to say, the dietitian wasn't too crazy about me. I could tell by her general attitude and lack of concern for my problem that she had never been overweight. When I made the comment that she had obviously never been fat, she snipped, "We're not here to discuss my weight." The whole conversation made me sick. There was not the tiniest ounce of encouragement. Do it her way or die. Any other attempt would end in failure, my fingernails would fall off, and I would go blind. That's how she made me feel.

I hung up the phone and said, "Nuts to you. I am going to do it. I'm going to eat the good, wholesome foods God placed on this earth for us to enjoy. When I've lost enough weight to no longer be embarrassed, I'll get that doctor exam, and unless fruits and vegetables cause cancer, I'll be okay."

Monday, March 18, 1985
216 pounds

I had an eye-opening experience Saturday. My friend Sarah knocked at my front door. There she was in all her glory, at least 200 pounds of it. My eyes zeroed in, not on her extremely overweight body, not on her new, short haircut, but on the huge bag of cookies and extra-large bag of chips from which she was so blatantly eating! I'm sure I showed shock, partly for her new look, that of a big balloon with a pea for a head. (Why do so many fat women insist on shaving off their hair, their one chance at having some fluff around their face to soften the chubbiness?) I was also shocked at her obvious lack of discretion in eating such fattening junk food.

But the real eye-opener didn't come till later in the day, after I'd spent two hours shopping with her. The whole time, I observed her steadily munching away on her huge bags of goodies. She didn't try to hide what she was doing or act nonchalant. In front of everyone, she kept popping those sugary, fatty morsels into her ever-open mouth. I thought, "Oh Sarah, how can you do this to yourself? How can you openly display your out-of-control behavior for everyone in this store to see?"

Being fat myself, I was embarrassed to be with her. I didn't want people to lump us together as two shameless, fat overeaters. It was repulsive seeing her eat in such an obnoxious way! At that precise moment, my eyes were opened; I understood her behavior. She had no idea how enormous she looked. As simple as that. When she passed a mirror, she still saw the waspish-waisted, movie-star figure she had years ago, the body that had once earned her "best swimsuit" award in a beauty contest. She didn't know. She couldn't see how wide she appeared from behind. Even while standing directly in front of a mirror, she refused to see how years of gluttony had acutely misshaped her once feminine form.

I felt a deep sorrow for her in that instant. I knew that if she realized how dreadful she looked, she wouldn't devour volumes of junk food in front of everyone. Oh, she would continue to eat the addicting morsels, unless she were somehow able to grab control, but she would eat only in private, a "closet eater." The kindest thing I could do for her would be to take some pictures of her, enlarge them, and send them to her.

When I first viewed the fat-pictures that Allen recently took of me, I thought it had to be a mistake. I said, "I know

I'm fat, but not *that* fat. I mean, everyone's heard pictures can add ten pounds—but 150 pounds?'' Thank goodness I viewed my pictures *after* I'd lost some weight and was on my way down. Even then, it was ghastly, but what would I have done if I had been as fat or fatter than in those pictures? Why, my own morbid obesity made them nearly obscene! I had never before allowed Allen to take pictures of me that fat. It was devastating, but in my determination to never be anywhere near that fat again, I allowed my hideous weight to be documented.

Fat people and pictures mix about as well as water and oil. Fat people avoid pictures with a passion. I see someone with a camera, and I get all crazy inside. A terror creeps through my whole body, and I try to get out of the room as fast as possible. Let's face it, pictures are too brutally honest. If I can't escape some family shot, I make sure that I'm the one holding the baby or that I'm standing in the back line. Check it out next time someone hauls out the camera. All the fatties head straight for the rear or try to push someone else in front of them. And I absolutely hate it (I have to control the urge to throw the camera in the punch bowl) when some jerk, would-be photographer decides to take quick, candid pictures. Oh, please, not candid pictures, those horrible, unflattering shots where I don't have any warning to suck in my stomach, pull up my chin, stand tall, or—gross me out—pull my blouse free from one of my own fat rolls.

Friday, March 29, 1985
212 pounds

Oh, sad, sad entry. My heart aches for my whole fat family. I will be relieved the next time all my brothers and sisters get together. I won't be the fattest person there. Oh! Not to be the fattest! It will be tragic for whoever takes my place, but let them have it. They can grab the reins right out of my hands! I've held those dirty, rotten reins long enough. I'm tired of being ashamed of my looks and my out-of-control behavior.

Each time we have a family gathering, I swear to myself, "Rosemary, you will not eat one sweet thing while you are there. Do you hear me, girl?" But as soon as I see all the good food and get one whiff of chocolate whatever-it-may-be, my resolve melts like a cube of butter in a microwave.

Have you ever watched a cube of butter melt in a microwave? Nothing happens for a couple of turns around the carousel. Then suddenly, without warning, one side burps out the liquid gold, and the whole cube caves in, melting within seconds. Exactly like my resolve. Even I don't realize how weakened it has become until it suddenly collapses, and I nonchalantly take my first bite. I really do act nonchalant. I would be mortified to let anyone know I was ready to melt the food down and shoot it up, trembling, mouth watering in anticipation of the ecstasy ahead. However, if you eat nonchalantly through a *whole evening*, you would be amazed how much you can consume.

I hate being at those family gatherings, where everyone can see how patently out of control I am. I'm shamed by the volumes I consume in front of everyone, and also by my appearance before I eat one calorie. I can never express how horrible it is to sit around with overweight people and *look* like you belong, but *feel* as though you have no business being there. Surely, I haven't let my life get as out of control as these fat people surrounding me. Yet I'm the fattest of all!

Now, at last, I'm on the brink of escaping. I'm excited to hold my head high again, hold my head high and my tummy in. Ah, success! I can smell it not too far down the road. When I've lost fifty pounds, I'm sure at least one person in my family will be motivated to start dieting. It will be too horrible for any of them to actually be "fatter than Rosemary." How I would love to be the catalyst for my whole family to get their weight under control. We are an unusually talented and funny group of siblings. We could form our own comedy club based on the jokes that flow from a single family gathering. Of course, half of those jokes are about our fat experiences and problems. Laughing about our weight problems helps us all to relax—and eat one more cookie!

Monday, April 1, 1985
211 pounds

April first, but I'm no fool! I weigh less than I have in years! Yesterday, at a baby shower, I was fascinated by a very fat lady. She insisted on eating candy continuously throughout the evening. I mean it; I am sure she ate all night because I watched her all night. Her mouth was never empty. In fact, the only time she stopped eating the chocolates on the table in front of her was while she was eating a piece of cake!

After she left, another fat person commented, "I think she purposely ate in front of us all night to make us believe that she doesn't care how fat she is." But I *know* she cares. Somewhere, sometime, she has to deal with her self-hatred and disgust.

I told Allen about this eater when I arrived home. He believed she was trying to say, "Hey, man, I'm me! I'll do what I want, no matter how I look. If you don't like me the way I am, then too bad for you. Nobody tells me what to do!"

I know better. That lady was not eating out of control because she doesn't care or because she doesn't want anyone telling her what to do. That pathetic lady was eating out of control because she *is* out of control. A chocolate demon has her by the throat, and she cannot break the choke hold. I am sorry for her. I know the horror too well. I know that some part of her is screaming out for help.

Wednesday, April 3, 1985
212 pounds

I am thrilled to record that I did not once go off my diet during the past two weeks while preparing the food for my parents' fiftieth wedding anniversary celebration. Being in control of myself gave me an awesome sense of power! I didn't feel the least deprived, only proud of my ability to say no thanks. I almost felt proud of the way I looked!

Now, I'm not blind. The mirror tells me I'm still fat, but I'm no longer appalling. I don't have huge rolls sticking out. And I have a new goal. Allen calls it my 40/60 plan. I want to lose forty more pounds in sixty days. If I follow my own checklist, I can do it!

> *February 27, 1992. I would no longer advocate trying to lose weight that fast without the supervision of a doctor. I have since learned that there are some health risks involved in losing weight too fast. I now try to lose about two pounds a week.*

For the present time, I must keep foremost in my mind that it is critical to take time for me. Nothing else is as important. I must remember that I am not being selfish. I need a few more months for *me*; then I'll be able to give of myself and help others, especially my own family, in a way I never could as the shapeless mass I have been.

Allen started talking vacation yesterday. My eyes lit up, and a shiver of excitement ran through me. I have never been so eager for a vacation. In fact, for years the word *vacation* has brought with it a dark cloud of fear. Depressing thoughts repeatedly run rampant in my mind for weeks before we leave: "I don't have any decent clothes to wear. Can I join in any physical activities? Will I subconsciously pick fights with Allen to give me an excuse not to participate?" And the list goes on.

Talk of vacation has filled me with that horrid awareness

that I can't run on any beaches, swim in any pools, climb any hills, fit on any amusement-park rides. I must constantly worry about running out of breath or falling down and hurting myself, being too fat for anyone to lift.

By June, I will be down seventy pounds. So yesterday, when Allen mentioned vacation, I felt like a child contemplating Disneyland. This vacation I will have clothes to wear. I will be able to participate in any activity! I won't need to pick fights. I will be able to enjoy a fun time with my family—minus seventy pounds!

This forty-pound loss, this first third of the lard, has unlocked a door for me. I'm cautiously stepping out, eyes wide open and seeing the world as a whole, new person. I have been imprisoned for twelve years. It's splendid to be stretching my wings at last! Yesterday I noticed three men staring at me with smiles on their faces. Oh, wow! One of them was *my* man. Double wow! And this is just the beginning.

Thursday, April 4, 1985
210 pounds

Yesterday I was free. Today I am furious—with Allen! I ate and ate and ate. I wasn't hungry. I ate to "show Allen." Ha! I only "showed" I am a fool. I knew I was eating too much greasy chicken right before bed. I knew I'd be sorry. I woke up nauseated in the middle of the night. I can never describe the shame I feel at knowingly doing something so stupid. Just admitting it in my own diary is torture. Sometimes I feel as though I have to write about it as a way of punishing myself.

Friday, April 5, 1985
210 pounds

As a child, I had a feverish determination to *never* get fat. There was no sense to it, no excuse for it. I'd lived with fat people and seen what fat could do to relationships, fun activities, looks, everything. I would never allow it! I'd seen several relatives get fat when they had their first child; I was disgusted with their fat and was positive I would not do that to myself or my marriage—so I thought.

Oh, that insidious line: "It's okay, I'll take care of it tomorrow. I'll diet tomorrow. This is the last, I mean the very last, time I pig out. One more little candy bar can't possibly hurt me!" I kept that it-can't-hurt-me attitude till I'd blimped up to 263 pounds. One candy bar wouldn't hurt me. But I never could stop with one. (An addict is an addict!) Oh, what a spectacular virtue, that of self-control. Would that I had a half pound of it!

When I was growing up, I became pretty sick of hearing "Next week, I'm going on a diet" or "After Christmas, I'm going to start" or "After all, this is my birthday. I can have as much as I want of my own birthday cake." I heard it constantly throughout my childhood. That kind of rationalization seemed incredibly stupid to me. Why would any grown-up purposely plan ahead to overeat until a particular day? I mean, overeating is a problem, right? It is unacceptable to *plan* to do anything wrong. How stupid it sounds when applied to any other problem: "I'm going to quit lying in three weeks." "I'm going to quit stealing after Christmas." "This is my birthday; today I will tease my little sister unmercifully." Utterly absurd! Yet people *plan* to overeat!

When I heard those same, old, lame excuses for putting off dieting, I often thought, "Oh, please, if you're going to diet, just do it! Don't merely *talk* about doing it. If you'll really lose weight, everyone will notice anyway, and you won't have to say one word."

I have always been too chagrined by my size to tell someone "Tomorrow." Now, I've often told *myself* that. You know, the old "Just this one last fling. This one last affair with chocolate." Ha! I never thought I'd be disloyal to my husband by way of candy, but I'll bet that few people who cheat on their spouses are more clever, deceitful, or guilty than I.

Oh, yes, I've lied to myself many a time, but I've always been guarded about committing myself to others. Even this time, when I *knew* I was doing it—I am going all the way down to 125 pounds—I held off saying anything until people started to notice. It's foolish to broadcast your likely failures to others. If you can click into gear and go on a diet, do it, but avoid embarrassing others and yourself with grandiose promises you both know will likely be broken.

Of course, Allen has heard more about my weight than anyone. My tears, self-hatred, and promises have been common occurrences for him. Yet even he has no idea of the depth of my past misery.

Just as I thought *I* would never get fat, I would have felt safe in betting money that my sister Rebecca never would, either. It was no gamble. It was a sure thing. She was beautiful. She was skinny. She never passed a mirror or a window or a piece of aluminum foil without brushing her hair or putting on more makeup. There was one word for her—glamorous! She was constantly singing the words to "Hollywood," and she looked like she was bound for the place. Everywhere she went, she'd declare with a toss of her head, "I just know some Hollywood producer will be here and discover me!" No, Rebecca would never get fat.

But many years ago, Allen told me she would. He said no one could eat that much candy and keep a decent figure. "It will catch up with her someday." Poor Rebecca. It caught up with her and grabbed her by the throat and is shaking its head like a dog with a rat in its mouth!

Rebecca called me a few days ago to ask about the Girl Scout cookies she had ordered from Jennifer. "If they've arrived and you bring them over *right now*, I'll buy some extra boxes." Oh, Rebecca! What a tragedy. Didn't she realize how pitiful, how desperate she sounded? Couldn't she see how pathetic her request was—asking me to quickly deliver the goods in order to instantly satisfy her addiction?

We human beings are capable of designing technology that can do almost anything. How can we allow our urges for sweets to control, even devastate, our lives? When I told Rebecca the cookies had not yet arrived, she said, "That's okay. I have the truck. I can go get some M&M's." And I once thought she would never get fat.

In fact, she was voted best figure in high school. She knew she had a pretty good chance at winning that coveted award, so she didn't eat a single bite at her senior-class breakfast. She was wearing a form-fitting dress, and if she had eaten one bite of sausage, you would have seen the outline of it on her tummy! But that was in 1974.

Yesterday, Rebecca called again to see if the cookies had arrived. In her own, unique, recite-the-dictionary-in-one-breath way, she blurted out, "If you bring over my cookies right now I'll buy a few extra boxes but it's no big deal 'cuz I can send one of my neighbor's children to the store and I see the neighbor girl across the street and she's selling the most sensational chocolate bars!" I felt sick that Jennifer had asked Rebecca to buy cookies that in any way contributed to her addiction to sweets. (But then, why should M&M's get all the business?)

I hope that somehow my weight loss will motivate her. Rosemary has always been the fattest. My sisters could be comfortable in their little thirty-fifty-seventy-five-pound overload because Rosemary would top any of them. Well, no more! I'm eighty-five puny pounds from perfection, fifty pounds from looking pretty good. And who knows? When my sisters can no longer subconsciously use my humongous size as an excuse to overeat, they might get motivated to lose weight themselves. I would be thrilled to be their reason to *think diet*, instead of being their excuse to *deep-fry it*.

Last night at the children's school carnival, a sort of magic happened. I experienced a fairy-tale euphoria. When you're losing weight, you don't measure time by days or weeks; you measure it by the pounds you've lost. When I told Allen, "I see people here who haven't seen me for forty pounds," he got a real kick out of it. And, brother, so did I. I felt like a celebrity. People were staring at me! It was a monumental moment. Some gave me the thumbs-up sign of approval. Several came up and told me I looked great. It was a paradox. I felt petite. Two hundred ten pounds, and I felt petite!

Tuesday, April 9, 1985
210 pounds

If I hear one more obese person whine to me that she doesn't have the money for diet foods, I will scream at her. I will unmercifully spit out the truth: "Who do you think you are fooling here? It's me, Rosemary. I know all the tricks, remember?"

Exactly what are you eating, pray tell, to maintain your bulk? The price of one single candy bar would provide the money needed that day for a package of Sugar Free Jell-O, or a couple of diet pops, or a piece of chicken, or a head of lettuce, or vitamins. And I know better than to believe that one single candy bar a day is making you that fat! You have to be spending a lot of money on mega-amounts of your favorite foods. No, lack of money is not the issue with a fat person. It takes dollars, bread, cash, dough, to maintain that ponderous bulk.

In fact, one of my worst nightmares is that people could somehow know how much I eat each day. You know, as if I had one of those cartoon bubbles above my head showing all that I'd consumed in the last twenty-four hours. Yikes! Of course, in a way, you *can* see all I've consumed.

Sometime ago, I barely survived another of my worst nightmares. My feelings of that day are as vivid as ever. I am once again in Mervyn's, talking over a purchase with my daughter Jenny, when suddenly I see . . . an old boyfriend. Oh, humiliation and remorse! Oh, self-hatred and "Please,

God, let the floor swallow me up!'' Oh, try to hold up my double chin. It was the longest two minutes of my life. I would rather clean all the bathrooms at the bus station than have *him* see me like this. This . . . this 250-plus-pound blubberball that can't even button up her huge coat. I looked exactly like what I had become: a fat housewife.

I felt as if only I were frozen in time. Everyone around me was moving. I couldn't think. I could hardly breathe. I wanted to cry. I wanted to scream.

I was furious with myself for not taking the time that day to look the best I could. At least then I feel like a classy fat lady. But that day, I felt every second my age and every ounce my weight! He didn't try to talk to me. (Thank goodness, because I might have thrown up on him!) Believe me, I made sure we did not make eye contact. But I felt his eyes on me. I knew it was him, and with a sideways glance I could see that he recognized me. I would have loved to walk over and say ''Hi, Ron.'' Ours had been a sweet, teenage love, and I have fond memories of our innocent relationship. But I couldn't say hi. I just couldn't. I lost my freedom in matters of that kind about fifty pounds ago. No, I had to pretend I didn't see him. Another victory for blubber.

Friday, April 12, 1985
207 pounds

What a glorious solitude! I sit here on the sand of Ocean Shores, Washington, with my toes digging into the moist softness, the gentle breeze blowing my hair and my writing paper, and the majestic waves rolling in, over and over like the sweet, soothing tune of a baby's lullaby. Even my poor, little, sand-stranded car, which I rest against, can't depress me. The world is mine, created especially for me, with all its glories and miseries, triumphs and failures, heavens and hells.

Ah, I have fought the good fight—and I have won! There

is still penance to pay, but the war is over! Never again will I have to risk life or limb for a piece of cheesecake. Never again will I need to venture into hell's mouth for a chocolate candy bar. Never again will I need to take the chance of losing children and husband to a cream puff. The war is over. Never again will anything be like this. This hell of my own making, this self-destructive, miserable experience of "pigitis." I thank God daily, almost hourly, for helping me, for throwing me the rope, the lifeline to freedom, before it was too late!

Today I was going to go horseback riding for the first time in years. Me! Two hundred seven pounds of me. I am almost human now. I was anxious to taste life again. I'm sure Allen didn't *try* to get the car stuck. A sign on the beach read: NO CARS BETWEEN POST AND OCEAN. Ah, come on, Allen, there were three million car tracks between the post and the ocean. But would he drive on the wet sand? Noooo! He had to obey the rules and get us stuck. That man is so honest, he'd get flustered lying to get someone to come to their own surprise birthday party!

The whole experience was rather funny. I was disappointed I didn't get to go horseback riding, though. My first big stab at real life, thwarted. But it's okay. I have years ahead of me!

It was all too symbolic as we were trying to push our car out of the sand. It was as hard to move our car as it is to get this fat lady to go on a diet. Someone threw us a rope and towed us to freedom that day. I've also caught *my* rope, and though the climb is steep, catching the rope was the hardest part! Oh, wouldn't it be wonderful if fat people everywhere could somehow grab on to the rope and be pulled out of their misery? I want to offer them the rope I've made myself. A rope woven of blood, sweat, and tears from the last thirteen years.

January 16, 1991. I have learned much in the long years since I made that presumptuous statement: ". . . but the war is over!" The sad truth is that

*this war will never be over for me—or people like
me. Obesity is an addiction that we must fight every
day for the rest of our lives.*

Friday, April 19, 1985
206 pounds

I feel like Gene Kelly when he sang "Gotta Dance!" in that
enchanting musical, *Singin' in the Rain*. I know how he feels.
I gotta write. I mean, I *have* to. Extraordinary feelings and
thoughts have been welling up in me for a week now, and I
can hardly stand it. This week, my goal was to get my desk
cleaned off. I decided it was necessary to *find* my diary before
I could write in it!

Writing is the ultimate way to express myself. Thoughts
that I don't recognize as my own sometimes come from my
pen. It's interesting to find hidden facts and feelings about
myself. Whenever I write about dieting, it makes me feel
recommitted. Then my soul craves to do all the things on my
Daily Checklist.

Saturday, April 20, 1985
205 pounds

Ah-ha! Another pound. One more fat, ugly bulge! My first
reaction was, "Oh! Big deal. One pound. I started out with
125 pounds to lose. What's one pound, more or less? A
tablespoon of butter?" Then I thought seriously: "Wait a
minute—what *is* one pound? It's a lot more than one tablespoon of butter." Let's see, there are eight tablespoons in a
stick, and . . . wow! I lost four sticks of butter yesterday!
Four hunks of lard! I am talking greasy fat here, not toned-
up, firm, beautiful human flesh. I'm talking the greasy, slimy
stuff that cooks out of your beef and ham roasts, then turns
hard and white when chilled. I'm talking about the pound of

grease you drain off hamburger and throw away. I'm talking about the layer of oil on top of soups that must be ladled off and discarded. I mean, no one wants it. Fat is ugly, dead or alive! And yesterday I ladled off one whole pound of it.

Something has happened inside me that surprises even me: Losing weight has almost enabled me to regain my youth. I've felt like an old grandma for too many years, simply because action has been out of the question. Fat has immobilized me, denied me entrance to many activities. Let's face it, bouncing blubber is hideous and disgusting, and I have the right to say that because I'm fat, and my blubber bounces!

But two nights ago, I experienced a little freedom from fat. I had a wonderful experience with seven-year-old Matthew at a Cub Scout pack meeting. It all started with Old McDonald, the one with the farm. When my group had to sing "with a 'moo moo' here and a 'moo moo' there," I didn't die the thousand deaths. I didn't take it personally. I didn't hate the Cub master, the whole meeting, or even my son. Do you understand yet? Forty-five pounds ago, it would have been miserable; now it was fun. When they asked mothers to come up and participate, who jumped up first? Me! Two hundred six pounds of me, not 250-plus.

At 250-plus pounds, I would have sat there torturing myself with hatred—for me *and* them! "How dare they ask me to stand up in front of people and sing anything reminiscent of moo-moo? (The only thing worse would be to sing oink-oink!) And what other harebrained schemes do they have in mind for us? Will I have to make an even bigger fool of my fat self? They better not try to make me!"

What a difference forty-five pounds can make! Even at an obese 206 pounds, I quickly jumped up, ready to participate! As I walked to the front of the group, I thought, "So this is what it feels like to join in the fun! This is what it feels like to be free to do as I choose. It sure beats standing back, trying not to be noticed, trying not to move too fast or jiggle too much."

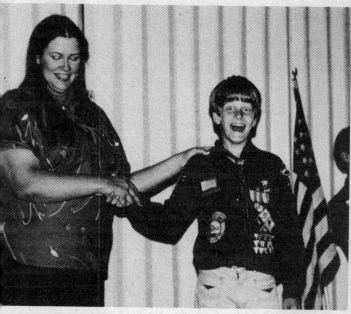

September 1983, 270 pounds. I was consumed with self-hatred at this weight. I was Cubmaster and had to conduct the meeting. Even as I awarded my son Jeremy his badges, I wanted to die with every breath I took!

Wednesday, April 24, 1985, 9:00 A.M.
203 pounds

Another pound! Four more sticks gone! Oh, every little piece of cake I didn't take, every sandwich I passed by, and every M&M I said no to—I don't miss you, I never will! My own strength is growing daily; it's as if my fat is somehow melting into resolve to lose even more. The lower my weight, the greater my willpower.

In my wildest dreams, I hadn't planned on the elation, this lift-me-off-the-ground sensation, of this weight-loss experience. Only by suffering the acute misery of fat could I appreciate this intense joy of release. Acquaintances are staring at me everywhere I go. They're thinking, "She's losing weight. Wonder how far she'll go. Wonder how soon she'll put it back on." I am determined to show 'em all!

Last night I had an exhilarating experience. I have written before in my diary, "I do have some fine, even noble ideas, and I will yet have my day in court." Well, last night it happened. A tiny bit of magic—a magnificent and terrifying moment. I attended a middle-school band recital. The parents were in the front seats of the auditorium and student-participants in the rear seats. I was disgusted and angry with the behavior of those students. It was unbelievable. If their rudeness had taken place during the intermission, it would have been inexcusable, but this loud, obnoxious behavior was taking place during the performance itself!

These twelve- and thirteen-year-old students were talking, laughing, shoving, moving, throwing, and snickering while other students were performing! It frightened me when I realized what that meant. Think about it. Parents were in the audience while these youths were behaving abominably. What were these same youths like in school, where no parents "dared to go"? That is a scary thought.

A total of nine school bands were participating. After sitting through the performances of the first two bands, with the young people as rude as could be, I was raging inside. I didn't have to put up with it! I marched to the middle aisle, faced those smarty little punks, and had my first "day in court." I had my first opportunity as a getting-thinner person to express myself openly. With all the expertise of a seasoned director of plays, I used my stage voice and could be heard throughout the whole auditorium, sans microphone: "There is absolutely no excuse for the rude behavior that has been displayed here tonight! You are middle-school children, but you've been acting like ill-mannered preschoolers. After listening to their children practice for hundreds of hours at home, all these parents have come tonight to hear them perform. How dare you make it impossible for us to hear the music? How dare you? Shape up and behave yourselves—right now!''

Oh, the fury that raged within me. The thrill of being in control of a situation, of myself. And, quite frankly, it was fun to have an audience. (If that doesn't sound like a frustrated, desperate actress!) I made my exit with an abrupt turn, to the thundering applause of the astonished but supportive parents.

When I returned to my seat, Allen put his arm around me and said, ''Good for you! What ever gave you the nerve to do it?'' The answer literally sprang to my lips, without forethought, unbidden. My eyes narrowed as I almost spat out, ''Forty-six pounds!''

Wednesday, April 24, 1985, 12:50 P.M.
203 pounds

I am delighted and shocked at the same time. My sister Rebecca called me this morning, and in the course of the conversation said, ''I heard you've lost forty-six pounds. With seventy-nine to go, you have less to lose than I do. I need to lose eighty-one to reach my dream weight of one-fifteen.'' Yessss! I swear I was suddenly seven years old again, repeating that old childhood taunt, ''My dog's bigger than your dog!'' Only I was dancing and chanting, ''Becky's fatter than I am! Becky's fatter than I am!'' It was a great moment. An even better moment will occur at the next family gathering when it's obvious I am not the fattest sister anymore. No! Never again.

I was abruptly brought back to the here and now when Rebecca queried, ''Now, really, if you never lost any more weight, wouldn't you feel happy at the weight you are?''

Shocked by her question, I responded, ''Oh, no. I'd be miserable. I'm not as disgusted with myself as I used to be,

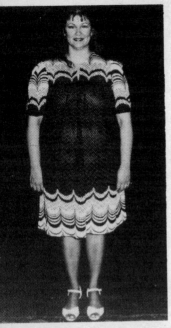 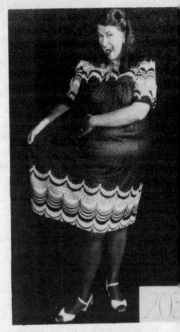

January 1985, 253 pounds, and April 1985, 203 pounds. Yes, I was elated with my weight loss. Who wouldn't be? Look at the difference!

especially because I'm on my way down. But I'm not kidding myself, either. I am still extremely fat."

"Well, I'm happy," Rebecca countered. "When I weighed one hundred seventeen pounds, I had to worry about every bite I took. Now I eat whatever I want."

At this point, my mouth was hanging open with disbelief. I'm glad that even through my years of morbid obesity, I have been able to be honest with myself. I have hated with a passion every pound, every ounce of extra fat on my body.

I replied with frankness to Rebecca, "Well, *I'm* certainly *not* happy. I just viewed some pictures of myself at my present weight, and it was a nightmare. I look like the star of *The Blob*!"

May 4, 1991. Rebecca obviously wasn't all that thrilled with her excess weight, after all. She hit the diet big time, and less than twenty-four months later, she was down to that miserable 117 pounds where she had to worry about every bite she took. Believe me, she didn't bemoan the trials of being a size five! I never once heard her express a desire to be extremely obese again, never once heard her complain that she could no longer eat a quart of ice cream each night.

Wednesday, May 1, 1985
200 pounds

Writing is the most satisfying activity of my personal time. It was an elating discovery to find out I even like me. When I write, I can separate the me from all the dumb, unaccountable things I do; I can sort through all the dirt to the seed of truth, to the speck of goodness that is my real heart and soul. When I write, I can feel that little seed shake and squirm to unleash the power within. Someday, that seed will send up a beautiful flower. Someday, I will emerge, not only from this ugly fat shell of flesh, but also from the sometimes stupid, thoughtless, and lazy ways I have come to accept of myself—and be the me I am capable of being. What a day that will be.

I've mentioned The Rose Festival before in my diary, but I have never fully explained what it is. The Rose Festival is to Portland, Oregon, what Disneyland is to Anaheim, California. It's two weeks every June, full of fun activities, parades, races, and contests.

Being chosen a Rose Festival princess in Portland is like

being Miss America in the United States. It's *hot stuff*. In fact, in June, I'm sure Rose Festival princesses are more easily recognized by Portlanders than Miss America would be. Their pictures are everywhere. One Rose Festival princess is selected from each Portland high school. And, yes folks, this incredible hulk was once a Rose Festival princess: beautiful, size ten, graceful, a real knockout! I may be fat, but I'm *not* blind. When I compare my present reflection to my pictures from fifteen years ago, I am shocked at what that beautiful young girl has become. Fifteen short—long—years. In my worst nightmare, I never imagined I was capable of becoming so obese. Or that my life could be such self-inflicted hell.

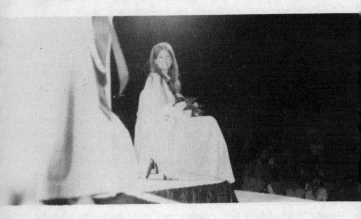

June 1970, 142 pounds. Yup, I could handle looking like a Rose Festival princess again!

Yet once upon a time, I was a Rose Festival princess. There were thirteen princesses chosen that year. We were honored at breakfasts, luncheons, dinners. We were showered with clothes, shoes, jewelry, cameras. We visited zoos, amusement parks, government buildings, hospitals. We were introduced to mayors, the governor, veterans, famous people.

We laughed, spoke, sang, entertained. We were treated royally and momentarily felt like honest-to-goodness, blue-blooded princesses.

Then it was all over. We came back to reality and went about the business of growing up. All thirteen princesses had recently graduated from high school. I was the first one to get married, the first one to have a baby, *and* the first one to get fat.

Each year, there is a special reunion of all the past Rose Festival courts. I remember my feelings distinctly in 1970, when ours was the reigning court, the one in the spotlight. I was seventeen at the time. I looked around at all the "old" Rose Festival courts, thinking my intolerant, seventeen-year-old thoughts: "Oh, look how old some of the ladies are. How could that fat lady come and let everyone know she's gone to pot? How could she ever have done that to herself? How could she ever live with herself?"

Yes, folks, those very thoughts ran rampant through my mind that night when I was young. When I was beautiful. When I was thin. When my skin was perfect and my hair thick. When I was seventeen. And that is exactly why I can no longer go to the Rose Festival reunions. I cannot sit there knowing some seventeen-year-old is thinking the same thoughts about me.

And so, I haven't gone since 1976. Oh, the ache, the humiliation of it. I am not free to choose. It's beyond me. I *can't* go. I have lost my freedom in the matter. I once memorized a phrase as a carefree youth, not realizing the depths of its poignant reality:

> "Of all sad words of tongue or pen
> The saddest are these, 'It might have been.' "

At our court's first reunion, I was eighteen, married three weeks. I attended that one. At the time of the second reunion, I was five months pregnant but looked full-term and then some. And I was carrying the baby so high—you know, in my upper arms and around my throat! Needless to say, I didn't appear at the reunion that year. Or at the next three.

The first of June 1976, Jennifer was eight months old. I'd just lost 33 pounds, bringing me down to a paltry 183. It was hard to get up the nerve to go. I was a full forty pounds heavier than I was as a Rose Festival princess. But with Jenny in one arm, trying to convince myself that she could hide those forty pounds (what a laugh), I ventured forth. My second and last time. Two out of fourteen. The other twelve times, I couldn't face the scrutiny of that roomful of beauty-contest winners. And *no way* could I face the girls from the 1970 court—the girls with whom I had laughed and primped and danced and sung. My court. My year. I couldn't put myself through that kind of torture. No, better to stay away and let them think what they wanted.

The hideous misery of my obesity, of all obesity, makes me sob. My out-in-the-open-for-everyone-to-stare-at lack of self-control is the ultimate tragedy. It's been a cruel punishment for eating too many candy bars. All the other girls on our 1970 court had encountered a variety of problems; they, too, had no doubt made serious mistakes. But I couldn't go . . . because I'm too fat. Some of their sins may have been more grievous, but mine was more obvious, more outwardly obnoxious.

Last winter, I met one of the girls from my court while shopping. There she was—110 pounds tops. I was almost two and a half times her size, weighing over 260 pounds. We talked a few minutes. I would have given anything at that moment to have the earth swallow me up so that I could cease to exist. Not just die. I wanted to *cease* to exist. I wished I had never been. That no one or no thing had ever been. Do you understand? I wanted blackness, nothingness, no one. I wanted everything to just be . . . gone.

It helped a tiny fraction to have Allen and my four children there. I wanted to scream out; "See, he has stayed with me—I must be worth something. Look at my four beautiful children. You bony, waspish-waisted, never-known-what-it-is-like-to-be-great-with-child model, I have some excuse for my monstrous size! So I gained 'a few pounds' with each baby.''

Somehow, I managed to survive that five-minute conversation. But then—oh, cruelest question of all: ''Why don't you come to the next Rose Festival reunion?'' My heart nearly stopped right then and there.

In a split second, all the hurt from the years of missed reunions, missed friendships, missed fun, missed life itself crowded in on me, and these thoughts rushed involuntarily into my mind: ''Yeah, well why don't you go to . . . go to . . . go eat a Twinkie? Which half of me shall I bring? Which one of my size-twenty-four-and-a-half dresses shall I wear? Which roll shall I try to hide with my folded arms? Why don't I come to the next Rose Festival reunion? Oh, get real! You know good and well why I won't be there! You probably all sit around and discuss where so and so is and what happened to her. 'She got really fat.' Do you think I don't know? Do you think I don't care?''

Saturday, May 4, 1985
203 pounds

Even at my current 203 pounds, I could never go to a Rose Festival reunion. But next year I'm going. And I'm going to hire a drummer and trumpeter to give me a drum roll and a *da-da-da-daaaa-da-daaaa* as I enter. I'll hire a footman to roll out a long, red carpet. I'm going to wear a gown that would put the ballroom scene from *Gone With the Wind* to shame.

But getting back to reality, to the 203 pounds of now. My darling, bubbly Jennifer was chosen a Junior Rose Festival princess on April 10. One hundred and twenty-one girls tried out from about fifteen different elementary schools. Oh, how proud I was. I was much more delighted for her as a princess than I'd been for myself. I was also much more nervous. I'd been sick to my stomach all day. Then suddenly, the curtains opened, and there she was, seated on a white throne, with an armful of gorgeous red roses. My beautiful little nine-year-old.

I went crazy. I was called up to the front of the auditorium to fill out information forms. With each step I took, each inch closer I came to the front, I was thankful for every one of the forty-six pounds I'd lost. I was still obese, but what a difference! I don't know what I would have done rolling down the aisle at 260-plus pounds. I don't think I could have endured it. Especially since Jennifer's talk mentioned that I'd been a princess in 1970.

Many people asked me about being a senior princess and thought it was neat that we had both been chosen. (Yes, thankful for each hideous little pound of greasy lard that was gone!) Then we had to hurry to *The Oregonian*, where Jennifer had her picture taken. She was darling! What a smile. I was questioned about my own experience as a Rose Festival princess, and then—horror of horrors—they asked to take a picture of us together! (We're talking thankful beyond belief here!) I was still mortified, sitting there with my fat bulging around me. But if I hadn't lost those forty-six pounds, I probably would have stopped breathing. Let's be honest; I would have refused to have my picture taken!

And later? When the parents were invited to the first official gathering of the eight junior princesses? I was intensely relieved when I saw I wasn't the fattest mother there. I didn't have to crawl into a corner, wanting to die. I didn't have to sit in a chair the whole time and hold my purse in precisely the right position to hide as much fat as possible. I didn't have to frantically demand that Allen stand next to me, to be my link with normalcy. I could actually enjoy myself! I felt like a real person, not a walking, talking tub of butter.

But right now, this minute, I'm mad! I'm furious with this nincompoop that inhabits my body. My 40/60 plan! Ha! It started exactly thirty-two days ago, and I've lost a grand total of five pounds. This morning, I stared at myself naked in front of a full-length mirror. Yikes! It was a good punishment for my overindulgences of the past. It was distressingly evident that I still need to drop some major rolls!

Today is the day! This is it! My pen can't write fast enough. No more rationalizing with "I can have vegetables, so, why not deep-fried onion rings?" Because they're breaded and full of grease, you turkey! And you know it. Quit trying to kid yourself!

Another example of how I try to fool myself is when I'm fixing popcorn. I allow myself two tablespoons of margarine. But I purposely cut the stick at an angle, to get a little more of the buttery flavor. I know it's stupid, I know I'm getting a few more fat-filled calories that way, but I still do it! I say to myself, "This is only two hundred calories." Stupid, fatty me ignores the prick of common sense that tells me it's really 225 calories or more, because of the slant at which I cut the margarine. Can you believe that? Well, I've *had* it with me!

Watch out, world! I'm coming alive. I'm a baby chick pecking its way out of its shell, a dormant volcano about to erupt. I must go it alone. No one can do it for me. It must all come from within. Allen can support and encourage, but no matter how hard the coach works, no score is made unless the *player* carries the ball into the end zone. At this moment, I have the ball, and I see the goalposts, and I'm going to stop meandering toward them. I'm going to take off in a hot run and not stop till I cross that blessed white line!

Tuesday, May 7, 1985
203 pounds

Tomorrow is Jennifer's first official Rose Festival affair. It's free for her. Ha! Believe me, the cost of feeding eight little nine-year-olds is easily covered by inviting doting parents and grandparents at ten dollars a plate! Dad, Mom, and three grandparents are going. Fifty dollars! Wow. That's a lot of bucks. Anytime I lay out that much money for a meal, the tightwad in me immediately determines to eat every last bite of food that is placed before me. It is totally irrelevant whether I like it or not. I will be overcome with the need to scrape my plate clean! That's how I will feel! Doesn't matter if the food is completely off my diet; I paid for it, I'm going to eat it. That foolish line of reasoning is responsible for at least ten extra pounds I carry around as my constant companion.

I must commit myself to myself in writing before I go to the luncheon tomorrow. No matter what is served, ten dollars is much less important than sticking to my diet.

Thursday, May 9, 1985
200 pounds

It worked! Writing in my diary really worked. I protected myself by thinking ahead. I turned my good intentions into a commitment by writing them down. I was able to stay in control. I'd lost fifty pounds and earned the right to eat any fruit I wanted. The fruit cup was manna from heaven. I gave the rolls, the rice, and the dessert to Allen. I am feeling so dedicated. So *magnifique!* I felt smug sitting there, almost cute.

Then I excused myself to use the rest room. Oh, curse you, full-length mirrors! You cruelest of all man's inventions. How dare you tell me the truth about my fat and insist on honestly displaying my 200-pound body for all the world to see? You dirty, rotten, nasty full-length mirrors. Needless to say, I was a little less than smug when I walked back into the banquet hall.

Yesterday, I exercised. There's a bit of a miracle in exercising, even when you're fat. It's invigorating and motivating. It helps me keep my diet in mind, and crazily enough, it enables me to *feel* my weight loss. When I put my hands on my hips and lean sideways, I *feel* where the rolls used to be. When I sit and stretch forward to touch my toes, I can tell I'm stretching farther, easier. A little credit goes to the fact that my body is limbering up. But mostly, I can bend farther because there is less lard around my middle; some of the "shortening cans" are no longer hanging around my waist. I can see and *feel* the difference. Although I continue to find it horrible to face each new exercise session, when I am through with the ordeal, I feel invigorated and proud of myself for following through with something!

Saturday, May 11, 1985
199 pounds

One hundred and ninety-nine pounds! I weigh in the one-hundreds. I weigh in the same hundreds as my husband. I weigh in the same hundreds as when I was married and when I was Rose Festival princess. I weigh in the same hundreds my final goal is in. I can breathe a sigh of relief. I can hold my head a little higher. I am only seventy-four pounds from perfection. I have only eleven pounds to lose to be halfway to my goal. I have reached my first milestone. For me, fifty pounds was ultra-important. And I did it. Never, ever again will I have to contend with that disgusting fifty pounds. Never, ever again—if I'm nine and a half months pregnant with quintuplets—will I weigh in the two-hundreds.

I actually saw a waist today. When Allen put his arms around me, he said he felt curves. Curves! I'm almost a woman again! Everyone is commenting now. It's almost embarrassing, but I love it—people calling me "skinny" and lots of other soul-satisfying names. At 199 pounds, though, it is rather preposterous.

My sister Debbie desperately wants to lose thirty-three pounds. She asked me to call her every day to keep her dieting. I know how she feels. It's critical to have a "buddy," but I cannot help her at this time. Right now I must concentrate on me. At this moment, I'm my own guinea pig (with little "guinea" and lots of "pig"), and I can't share my program till I've reached my final goal.

It's fun to talk diet. All my fat friends are interested! "How are you doing it? Are you getting professional help? Pills? Liquid diets?'' My answer is so simple, it's almost embarrassing!

"I'm doing what I know I'm supposed to do. (All fat people know what they should be eating. All America knows about the four food groups.) I'm just eating like a normal person.'' That's the answer, the true miracle in a nutshell. "Eat what you *know* you should.'' That eliminates all the junk foods: pastries, chips, candy, pop, etc. Many foods in their natural form taste good, are good for you, and are not too fattening. One can find a virtual feast in fresh fruits and vegetables alone. The variety is astounding. The problem is, most of us want to sugarcoat or deep-fry everything that grows.

> *September 17, 1991. So we have advanced a little from "the four food groups." Many new facts about food have come to light. This knowledge makes us better equipped than ever to reach our various weight-loss goals. Foods with high fat content are definitely "out." (I'm afraid people with high fat content are, too.) The success formula for weight loss always has been and always will be: Ingest fewer calories than you expend!*

I've also experienced some sad moments in my weight loss. Three days ago, I was talking with my good friend Kathy. She has seen me weigh anywhere from 150 to 263 pounds. We've been up the scale together. She's had a weight problem, too, but never as serious as mine. I haven't seen her for at least eight months. I called her when I lost thirty-two, thirty-eight, and forty-eight pounds. Each time I called, she said she had gained more weight. Five days ago, I told her I was teetering at 200. When she reported being at her all-time high of 190 pounds, I exclaimed, "What do you know? I'm two inches taller than you, so we probably look about the same.''

Her immediate response? "Oh, no! I carry my weight

unusually well. I'm sure I look much better than you.'' Gee whiz! I needed a little praise from her. I wanted her to be happy for my success, even if she was furious with her own failure. I mean, how many times in the past had she said, ''Oh, Rosemary, I don't know how you can live with yourself. I'm so miserable, and you're *so* much fatter than I am.'' Now that I wasn't much fatter than she was, I wanted a wonderfully supportive response. But my success makes her failure more obvious, more hateful. It will kill her to weigh more than I do. It might even motivate her to start dieting herself. I hope so. And yet . . . the meany in me wants her to wait for a few more months. Wait till I weigh 125 and she weighs 190; then she'll have to eat her words instead of her cookies! Isn't that horrible of me!?

Two days ago, my sister Rebecca asked me how much more weight I wanted to lose. ''Seventy-five more pounds!'' I said it with a positive note in my voice. She responded, ''I need to lose sixty-five to be my perfect weight.'' Hmmmm. Only fifteen days ago, she told me she needed to lose 81 pounds to reach her dream weight of 115. It's interesting to me that she somehow ''lost'' sixteen pounds without looking any thinner. I suppose she, too, can't bear to be anywhere near the same weight as I am. She probably sees me as huge as ever in her mind and can't comprehend being anywhere near that size.

But in my mind, I'm 125 pounds. Running, swimming, biking, playing. The rest is ''clothing'' I must slowly peel off and say, ''See! It's me; I was here all along!''

Thursday, May 16, 1985
196 pounds

My daily exercising is becoming a reality because I have a regular time to do it each day. I turn on my answering machine as soon as I come home from taking the children to school and then . . . watch me huff and puff, twist and turn, grunt and groan. I really work up a sweat. Now, please don't misunderstand me. I do not delight in exercise. I do not look forward to stretching and straining. Getting out of breath is not my idea of a good time. To me, exercise is like medicine. Who wants it? But my body needs it! So I grit my teeth and take my shot!

Sometimes I envision the gorgeous, firm, fifty-year-old body of Jane Fonda. If I imagine myself sleek and svelte like Jane, I can then do one more curl-up. I see a lovely lady running in slow motion on the beach in a white swimsuit, and it's me, and I'm not jiggling! (At least not anyplace I'm not supposed to!) I have to envision that lovely lady in order to finish my leg lifts. In fact, the only thing that turns me on about exercising is that it feels so good to quit.

Friday, May 17, 1985
198 pounds

Once upon a time, there was a chubby little woman. One day, she decided to go on a diet. But, oh! It was so hard to tell exactly how much she weighed because her scale was not working terrifically. It could vary as much as eight pounds on the same day, at the same time, weighing the same person. Of course, this woman would get frustrated because it was difficult—no, impossible—to tell precisely how much she had gained or lost each day. Oh, she knew she was losing weight: her clothes fit better, she looked thinner, and the scale definitely showed a downward trend. But the poor woman was still frustrated because she didn't know her true weight. Every day she told her husband that when they could afford it, they must buy a new scale.

And so it was that over and over again for about four months, this chubby woman's husband heard how badly they needed a new scale, preferably a digital scale, as they were reported to be more accurate.

So can you guess what the husband bought his chubby

little wife for Mother's Day? That's right—a nice, new, digital scale. Oh, the chubby little wife was happy. Oh, she was excited. At last, she could measure her exact weight loss. "Why, thank you, thank you, darling husband!" Then that silly, chubby woman made the dumb mistake of weighing herself on the scale, right there in front of everybody! Right there with all her clothes on. Right there, after she'd eaten a large breakfast. Oh, silly, stupid, chubby woman.

The new scale, the scale that was going to be more accurate and easy to use—yes, that very scale—displayed in bright red, neonlike numbers: 212 pounds! Now this woman went crazy. She went berserk. She made no sense at all! After those four long months of bemoaning her lack of a reliable scale, she irrationally pronounced, "I wanted to pick out my own scale. I didn't really want a digital. I didn't really need a new scale!"

The poor husband. What should he do? Hadn't he heard with his own ears how she needed this very gift? Now he heard his chubby little wife getting hysterical: "Just leave me alone. Get out of here. Oh, what a stupid present!"

The baffled husband was innocent. He couldn't possibly understand how depressing, frustrating, even suicidal, it feels to suddenly have "gained" sixteen pounds. It didn't help to get logical. The wife was beyond logical. She was well past rational. To be suddenly sixteen pounds heavier than expected—sixteen more ugly pounds to lose! Let's face it, the wife lost her cookies. Kicking the scale out of the way and slamming doors after her, this chubby wife flounced into her room, threw herself on the bed, and sobbed her chubby little heart out.

Now, in mild defense of this woman one must know that only moments before her husband brought his gift into the bathroom, she had been already close to tears. Oh, vanity! Just because she was losing her hair, she was letting herself get depressed. A few seconds prior to her husband's entering the room, her thoughts were, "Oh, great. I'm going to be a bald-headed fat lady." So those extra sixteen pounds were all it took to do her in.

It is still incomprehensible that she would act like such a jerk, but she did . . . I did. Yes, folks, surprise, surprise! *I* was that silly, chubby, thinning-haired wife. I did it. I swear, there is a direct relationship between the number of extra fat globules on my body and the number of times I emotionally bonk out each week. Words can't describe the high-pitched, hysterical voice I used. But trust me, it was one of my most ridiculous scenes. And believe me, I've been in some pretty ridiculous scenes. I'm afraid it won't be my last, but I sure hope it will be my worst.

Saturday, May 25, 1985
200 pounds

I haven't written for several days. I'm staying away from my diary with a vengeance. I'm punishing it. I haven't lost any weight for three weeks, so I'll punish it good!

Monday, May 27, 1985
198 pounds

I love (love, LOVE, *LOVE!*) to hug my husband. And my children. And my aunts and uncles and cousins and nieces and nephews—as I choose. But have I ever mentioned how much I hate (hate, HATE, *HATE!*) being hugged by some slight acquaintance merely because it is the "thing to do"? I go to a meeting or social at school or church, or I see someone whom I haven't seen for years, or I meet a relative for the first time . . . and whammo! A giant bear hug! Certain people seem to think ya' gotta hug 'em to adequately say hi.

As a big fatty, I hate to have semi-strangers put their arms around me and feel my fat rolls. So now you know; we fat people are aware that you can feel our fat rolls every time you hug us. And yes, we hate it. Be fair! You can see every fat roll and bulge on our bodies. Please, give us the right to say who gets to touch them or hug them!

How I pray that someday I won't have to worry about someone hugging me and feeling my fat rolls—because there will simply be no fat rolls left to find!

Thursday, May 30, 1985
198 pounds

Wow! I just read my whole diary. I like it. It is motivating, at least for me. I'd forgotten some of those feelings I've mentioned. Writing them down when they happened was essential; I could never reconstruct certain events and emotions exactly as they occurred. I'm glad I read those pages. I needed the boost.

Less than two hours ago, I committed the "ultimate" sin. What could that be, you wonder? I ate, *and thoroughly enjoyed*, a lemon-cream-filled Van Duyn chocolate. Ahhhh! I didn't eat it because I was hungry. I ate it out of anger . . . and because some jerk in my family had left it lying around!

I've felt myself weakening the last few days. Steadily dropping those ugly pounds is essential to continued commitment to dieting. That's why I was reading my diary. I need the support it gives me. Also, Allen has been radically inconsistent in meeting with me daily. I'm not blaming him for my obesity, but, boy-oh-boy, is his support crucial to me and my diet.

Rebecca said she is happy at her weight. I find that hard (hairline from impossible) to believe. But even if she is, I'm not. I'm miserable. I want to be svelte. I want to go swimming. I want to do exercises without hearing my own blubber slap against my body. Have you ever heard that ghastly sound? You are lucky if you have no idea what I'm talking about. It nearly causes me to retch with disgust. My stomach actually bounces against the top of my legs and slaps me when I run.

I need help! It's a little frightening that whenever I call upon God for any help, it seems I inadvertently awaken another force. Its influence is strong. I hesitate to say "the devil"; that sounds so fanatical. But the universe is full of opposing forces. And my firm belief in God compels me to accept the ugly reality of the devil.

Many times these past few weeks, I've been inclined to say my prayers. But I have put the thought quickly from my mind, thinking I would do so in a few minutes. The prompting has come like incessant little pinpricks, and yet I've ignored or put off each little poke. I must continually seek God's help through prayer. I will not allow myself to forget. I want to succeed.

Friday, June 14, 1985
199 pounds

What would be the craziest thing for a serious dieter to do? To purposely get pregnant, right? Guess what? You are looking at the craziest serious dieter of all time! Yes, folks, this lady has deliberately put smack-dab in her diet path the biggest stumbling block of all. But I am determined to weigh less than 170 pounds when I deliver this baby. That's 100 pounds less than when I delivered my last baby, 40 pounds less than when I delivered my first. For crying out loud, a baby seldom weighs more than eleven pounds. There is no reason for me to gain eighty-five, as I've done in the past.

> *February 6, 1991. I need to mention here one of the great tragedies of my life. I lost the baby near the end of June. A new and horrible experience. Yes, one learns from such things, but pain is a cruel teacher. The miscarriage left me devastated. It is a difficult thing to grieve for the loss of a baby who*

was never born. I had to believe that I would yet hold another infant in my arms. My darling Jon Tyler, born August 1986, exceeded my fondest expectations. I am grateful for him each and every day!

Tuesday, July 2, 1985
205 pounds

Oh! What a horrible entry to have to write. I'd rather clean out my garage. I'd rather eat liver! I'd rather sit through another showing of *Gremlins*. But I must hold my head high and take my medicine, for only then can I get better. I must admit it in black and white: I haven't written for two and a half weeks. I've been undeniably *off* my diet, and I'm gaining back weight.

Whenever I don't adhere strictly to my regimen, it's as if the floodgates burst open, and I pull out all the stops. I go berserk and deliberately eat as if I'm preparing for a thirty-day fast, destroying my body, my life, and my dreams. I am not capable of eating only one cookie or one chocolate or one piece of cheesecake. I am mentally deficient in the area of controlled eating.

Sunday, July 7, 1985
206 pounds

A few short weeks ago, I was so proud, so high on life, so *sure* I would never go off my diet. People are watching me. I've made these grandiose commitments to everyone about the 125 pounds I would weigh on December 1, 1985, and look at me—I've gained back ten pounds. That puts me at— oh, gag, not again!—206 pounds. Soon everyone will notice. I can fake ten pounds, but ten more than that will put me halfway back to my miserable, humongous past. Oh, I'm afraid I would want to end my life.

Everything is different now. When I weighed this much going down the scale, I felt like a cute thing. But as the pounds add up, as I creep back up the hell scale, I see myself more clearly for what I really am. I am fat. My stomach hangs out like the proverbial spare tire. There is nothing alluring, sexy, or desirable about me. I am obese, and I will get worse if I don't stop here.

I'm rededicating my life to diet. The most important thing right now is me. Not friends, church, children, or husband! This weight loss is my most important reason for living, existing, being, or doing for the next six months.

My obesity is like a huge, oppressive cloak that is taking away my freedom of movement. Our founding fathers knew that freedom was everything and fought fiercely to obtain it. Like them, I must win my freedom!

I have the ultimate program, the perfect key to success. I suppose I'm almost thankful for this regression. I was so *sure* I'd never fall off my diet. I'm shocked and don't understand how or why it happened. I need to start from block A and do it all over again.

Wednesday, July 17, 1985
206 pounds

Okay, okay, okay. So nobody's perfect. So I failed again. First thing this morning, I ate a small piece of chocolate cake with extra chocolate frosting on it. I didn't like it, and heaven knows I didn't *need* it, but I stuffed it in anyway. Fast as I could. I'm tired of hating myself, so I must master my mouth.

One little bite of cake this morning will make no difference in my weight, only in my emotional outlook. It won't make me any fatter, but watch out—that one little piece of cake, early in the morning, is the green light to go ahead and eat garbage all day. I already blew it, right? So I'll splurge just this "one last day." These ten pounds I've gained back are gruesome. Worse than being physically obvious, they are emotionally devastating. A simple five-pound loss will relieve my anxiety attack!

No one said life was going to be easy. Controlling any bad habit or compulsion is a lifelong pursuit. Getting started is often the hardest part, but staying power is also essential. I suffered from a false sense of security. I was *sure* I would never fail, never go off my diet. Ha! Everyone is capable of certain crazy and irrational actions. The secret is that we all must learn to endure to the end.

No matter how well you start out in any endeavor, if you stop short, you fail! I'm not stopping short. I've strayed and messed up, but I'm not through yet. I'll fail only if I quit trying.

Wednesday, August 7, 1985
207 pounds

I can't go on any longer. I am going totally berserk! I want to run away. From what? From me, I think. I want to escape the mean, out-of-control individual who inhabits this body. I want to escape this putrid excuse of a body. That doesn't leave me much that I like about me, does it? I don't like my spirit, and I hate my body. What else is there, for crying out loud? I don't like any of me right now. No, I take that back. I was just admiring the shape of the index fingernail on my left hand. Woooo! I like my index fingernail. Like with three million square inches of body covering I should be ecstatic because I like one one-millionth of it. Well, it's a start. I don't understand how I can get so depressed. I am so low, I have a hard time lifting my shoulders to take a deep breath. I'd better quit writing.

Sunday, August 18, 1985
205 pounds

It's amazing to me that any human being has such resilience. There has to be more bounce-back ability in me than in a Super Ball. In fact, I feel as if I've been pumped full of flubber, the invention of an absentminded professor in a Walt Disney movie. Flubber was a fantastic discovery that produced its own energy. Each time it bounced, it progressed higher. Ah, yes, today that is how I feel! Yesterday I hit a new low, but with the sweet balm of sleep and the help of some inspired writings of Louisa May Alcott, the flubber principle in me has been unleashed, and today I am up, up, up! I've bounced higher than ever before.

The potential in me is about to burst forth. I feel my talents massing together, ready to attack any ugly, discouraging thought or person (or the devil himself) that might try to barge (or sneak) in and destroy me. I am going to use this "flubber" high to help me get rid of my blubber lows. In all honesty, most of my problems, failures, and miseries are a direct result of the "blubber blues."

Poor Allen is distraught trying to figure me out. I'm amazed that his sanity has lasted even half of the fourteen years we've been married. Sometimes I wonder if some weird little brain cell in my head is trying to see how long Allen will last, how hard I can push him. I love him so; I cannot comprehend how even one tiny brain cell would go awry.

Saturday, August 31, 1985
210 pounds

Why did husbands ever have to be invented? Most of the time, one could get along quite nicely without the nasty little creatures. Sometimes I look up into the heavens and ask, "Really now, God, why did you create rats . . . or head lice . . . or fleas? Why?" Well, at this moment I question the virtue or value of another disgusting menace to ultimate happiness in life: men—and in particular, husbands.

February 12, 1991. I tore half of the above entry from my diary at this point. I'm glad I destroyed it. I love my husband intensely, and, basically, he's been a jewel to me. I am sorry and shamed as I read my own comments about him. Many of them aren't fair.

Wednesday, September 18, 1985
212 pounds

Oh boy! Can I dream! I could get paid for my dreams! My biggest dream at present? I want to stick to my diet today. Grand dream, for not only do I want my freedom from fat, I want to publish this diary and my poetry book, be on Johnny Carson's *Tonight Show*, become Mrs. America, travel the world lecturing on weight loss, *and* be able to quit baby-sitting. Hopefully, not in that order.

However mundane, providing day care has enabled me to stay home with my own precious children. But I can't deny that I'm going Looney Tunes! I think a person has the capacity to change only a limited number of messy diapers in one lifetime. I am firmly convinced that I am reaching my limit. It's hard to think about, let alone write about, all my glorious dreams, with a dirty diaper in one hand and a baby washcloth in the other. Each time I change a diaper, wipe a nose, clean up a spill, wash fingerprints off the wall, trip over a toy, or hear the eternal "Rosemary, she hit me!" I will tell myself: "Diet, diet, diet. Everything depends on my diet. It is the pathway to freedom from fat and from baby-sitting." I want the free time to be able to accomplish some of my dreams. I can do it. I *will* do it. I mean—I think I have only three dirty diaper changes left in me.

Thursday, September 19, 1985
210 pounds

Yikes! I've been officially off my diet longer than I was on it. I am extremely disappointed with myself. Nothing and no one is worth eating over. There are definitely times in our lives that are more stressful than others, but fat only adds to the stress. This all-consuming feeling of self-hatred and guilt is unbearable.

I hate the scale fiercely each day because it is always the bearer of sad tidings. I hate it, and then I chuckle to myself. How silly to hate the scale. It's my fault, but I want to blame anyone or anything for this blubber body. Maybe my toothpaste has too many calories! Maybe my deodorant works too well, and I'm full of liquid trying to perspire out. I mean, I'll blame anything!

After I weigh myself and curse the scale, I look in the mirror, the huge mirror that shows (gag) everything! Then I realize, who cares if I weigh 200-plus pounds? It doesn't matter what I weigh. It matters only how I look. If I weighed 110 pounds and looked like this, I'd still be disgusting. I guess I won't blame the scale anymore . . . I'll blame the mirror. *That's* where I look awful. Yeah, that's it. It's the mirror's fault!

You know what's hard? It's when you look at a morbidly obese person eating or trying to run or to bend over or simply standing in line at the store, and your stomach turns over and you say to yourself, ''Oh, I'm so embarrassed for her or him.'' Then you glance down and realize you look worse. That is *so* hard.

Of course, most of the time you're not that honest with yourself. Most of the time you pretend that you don't look nearly as bad as that other fat person. Your brain can trick you into feeling smaller than you are. You know how a skinny person can suck in his stomach? Well, sometimes we butterballs mentally suck in our *whole bodies*. If we walk a little taller, perhaps no one will notice the extra 100 pounds.

Sometimes it's the only way I get up the nerve to go into a 7-Eleven and buy five candy bars. I have to think thin first, to somehow pull it all in, to promise myself this is the last, the very last, positively the *last* time I will ever do this. And I go through that several times a week.

Monday, September 23, 1985
208 pounds

I was getting ready to pull out of my space in a parking lot when I noticed a lady coming out of a store with a package of cigarettes in her hands! Oh, how disgusting! I could feel my lip curl back in disdain. That woman was so addicted that she had to make a special stop at a convenience store to satisfy her craving. She wasn't buying anything else. She had to stop her car, get out, spend her money, and then watch it literally go up in smoke. How could she live with herself? It just made me sick. It just . . .

Then I looked down in my lap. I looked down at the sack in my lap. I looked down at the three candy bars in the sack in my lap. Three candy bars! Oh, how disgusting! I could feel my lip curl back in disdain. I was so addicted that I had to make a special stop at a convenience store to satisfy my craving. I wasn't buying anything else. I had to stop my car, get out, spend my money, and then watch it literally turn to pure fat. How could I live with myself? It just made me sick.

Yes, folks, that day I learned to measure myself by the same yardstick I measure others. It was a good lesson. Smoking is a senseless, preventable health hazard. So is obesity. But at least smokers can get away from smoke from time to time. When is the last time you saw a fat person leave their fat behind? (Oops! That pun was unintentional.)

One more thought. That lady's pack of cigarettes probably lasted her the rest of the day. At least several hours. But my habit, my money sucker, was gone before I made it home from the store. Scary thought. Ha! Food for thought.

Tuesday, October 15, 1985
212 pounds

It's simply a matter of something clicking on in my head that finally gives me the courage and motivation to diet. An eminent religious leader of our day, Spencer W. Kimball, has a sign on his desk: DO IT. I can't think of any more sage advice to the obese person. For heaven's sake, "Just do it, just di-et"! And I *am* doing it.

All my fat cells are being refilled with weightless happiness. For every pound of blubber I lose, every greasy pound of disgusting lard I drop, I gain a pound of happiness. Okay, all you fatties out there. 'Fess up. Would you rather be carrying around enough butter to grease the Rose Bowl, or enough happiness to nearly lift you above the crowd? How would you like to be stared at for your broad smile instead of your broad hips? Wouldn't it be awesome to walk with your head held up by your pride of self, instead of by your triple chins! Dream with me for a moment, my fat friends, of walking with a charming little bounce in your step, instead of that disgusting bounce all over your body!

Something "clicked" in my head two days ago. I had been off my diet, in dark despair, since June first. I quit working my own program for success. My prayers, when they came, were heartfelt cries for help—from deep within: "Please, God, help me. I don't want to be fat. I'm gaining weight again. I'm terrified."

A week later: "Dear God, I'm here, don't leave me. I'm dying inside. I might kill myself. Life is too hard. I could not live at two hundred and fifty–plus pounds again. Stop me. Help me. Please, you're my only hope." The tragedy is, this kind of prayer was often uttered on the way to the store to buy candy bars.

Thursday, October 17, 1985
210 pounds

I feel like I've had my batteries charged for life. I've lost five pounds in the last four days. Life is fabulous when I'm in control of me.

I had been slowly climbing back up the hell scale. A few pounds here and there, the old lose-two, gain-three routine. I had gained back nineteen of the fifty-four pounds I'd lost. I felt so out of control, the best description of the feeling is one of drowning.

I did almost drown once, on a popular but dangerous beach near Sydney, Australia. I was helpless, vulnerable to the vicious current that attacked my body and slowly pulled me under, sucking the air out of my lungs, the life out of my body. I couldn't touch bottom, and couldn't keep afloat. As I gasped and choked, I thought, "This is it. It's all over. I can't make it to the surface for one more breath." Allen was by my side, but he could barely keep himself afloat.

"*Please*, I need only one good breath, just one gulp of life-sustaining air!" I pleaded silently. I was terrified. I was more than terrified. When you are as desperate for air as I was at that point, even terror is an understatement. Your whole being strains to do one thing—to live. I thought of my sister Joyce. She, too, had known the terror, the desperation. She drowned when she was fifteen. Ironically, I remembered in those moments that I am her namesake. I was named for Joyce Marie. And Joyce Marie had drowned. I clawed at the waves. *I had . . . to get just one . . . more . . . breath!*

And then, before I saw them, there they were. Angels of mercy. Two big, strong lifeguards—one at each elbow—pushing me up as each wave tried to crash over me. Pushing me ever forward toward shore. Moments later, as I lay on the velvety warm sand, all my feelings were acutely magnified. The sand was softer. The ocean was bluer. The clouds were fluffier. Life was dearer. I shall never forget lying on the shores of Bondi Beach, feeling thankful to be alive.

In a few minutes, when my emotions were back to normal, I was able to contemplate my brush with death. I hadn't known I'd been in danger until it was too late. *I hadn't even known.* I hadn't seen the sign right there on the beach. A clear-cut warning: BEWARE OF UNDERTOW! DO NOT SWIM BETWEEN TWO POSTS! Not seeing the sign did not erase the danger. The danger was always there. The consequences were just as deadly.

Many times since that scary day, I have thought, "How many signs in our lives do we so blithely pass by? How many warnings do we blindly skip around, then go on our merry little way?" Whether or not we see the signs, the danger is no less real.

For me, being obese evokes the same terror as drowning. When I can't get control, when I eat everything in sight and then think of what else there possibly is to cook or buy—when I can't touch bottom—it's then that I feel the waves crashing over me again, and I find it difficult to breathe.

"What will I do? My clothes are getting tight. People are noticing the gain. I can't be another statistic, another nameless face on the blubber express!"

Thursday, October 24, 1985
208 pounds

Even I cannot believe that after composing that dramatic analogy between the horrors of drowning and the horrors of overeating, I still could not quit shoveling in goodies like a trick-or-treater on Halloween. I cannot comprehend that I can lose sight of my glorious goal so easily. Show a little self-control, and joy and happiness reign. Give in to your physical desires, and misery takes over.

An important part of dieting is thinking thin. More than that, I have to dream and plan and imagine, to visualize myself with a trim waist, wearing blouses that (gasp) tuck in. It's those thoughts that keep me on my diet.

It takes dedicated time and effort to diet. Let everything else in your life suffer; nothing is as important to you as looking and feeling your finest, which leads to *doing* your finest. Neglect whatever you must. Cobwebs, dust, and clutter can wait. Let the children eat cold cereal and TV dinners, but take time for you. Eventually, when you're thin, you'll be much more productive and useful, a whole new person, and that will more than make up for any inconveniences suffered by your family while you were dieting.

It's essential to pray, write, exercise, look your best, and think thin. All these things take time. They must not be neglected. You cannot write while fixing dinner. If something must go, let it be dinner.

A week ago, I saw a newsclip on TV that made me sick. It showed five morbidly obese females discussing their weight. It was heart-wrenching, yet almost nauseating, just to view them! My whole being was overflowing with compassion for them. I knew their plight only too well—I had *been* one of them. But their attitudes were extremely confused. All of their conversation centered around the theme that "Big Is Beautiful." That philosophy is screwing up the minds of fat people.

"Big Is Beautiful," my eye! How many centerfolds have fat rolls hanging from their stomachs? Ripply, bulging thighs? Thick, fleshy necks, and the equivalent of a three-pound can of shortening dripping from each upper arm? Now, there is no one more opposed to pornographic magazines than I am. They are immoral and degrading to women. But even the insensitive monsters that publish such garbage recognize that fat is not beautiful. Fat does not sell magazines.

Let's not confuse "big" with "fat." A six-foot lady weighing 150 pounds would certainly be considered big, and, if she had a face like Jaclyn Smith, she would most definitely be considered beautiful. But I don't care what your face looks like, if you weigh 300 pounds, you definitely aren't beautiful. "Big" and "fat" are not synonymous. Big can be beautiful. Fat cannot. If I am so beautiful, why am I chagrined if my husband glimpses me stepping into the shower, or worse yet, into bed? What could be more degrading than trying to hide myself from the husband I sleep with? I hate writing this and facing these ugly facts!

You want to hear another cop-out excuse for out-of-control eating? These five appallingly fat people laid this one on thick: "Accept yourself for what you are." Oh, give me a break! In reality, that says: "Go ahead, eat like a pig, make yourself sick, deprive yourself of activities only thin people can enjoy, kill yourself off; it's okay."

I became enraged! What do they mean, "accept yourself"? For Pete's sake, why? What about the person who partially loses his hearing? Should he bother his friends and relatives by making them yell and constantly repeat themselves? Should he accept partial deafness? Or should he use a hearing aid? Similarly, fat is not acceptable! It's like telling your eye to accept a piece of dirt. It won't. The eye will wash the offensive intruder out with tears and get rid of it. Well, fat doesn't wash away. It goes with you everywhere. And it's not just irritating or uncomfortable—fat is ugly. It's ugly to wear and ugly to see. And I'm fat, so I can say that.

Even though fat poses a major impediment to beauty, it's important for every fat person to always *try* to look her best. It's inexcusable that so many fat people also have greasy hair, dirty fingernails, and torn clothing. Give us a break! Fat is bad enough by itself. Keep yourself clean and neat. Use makeup to enhance your facial features and draw attention to your face, not your body. Dress stylishly, but don't be fooled by those fashion designers and sales clerks who tell you to "break all the rules—*anyone* can wear a belt, ruffles on their hips, or humongous shoulder pads"!

What size-forty-four woman doesn't already have plenty of shoulder pads . . . permanently attached to her person? The fashion designers only want your money, and then they laugh behind your back. Really now, think about it: ruffles on size-forty-four hips? Naaaah!

Don't hate *yourself* for being fat; but do hate the *fat*. (That's a lot easier said than done!) Don't ever kid yourself into accepting your fat. Accept the fact that you have a problem.

But it is a problem that can be controlled. Always look forward to a better, thinner day. Don't kill yourself with self-hatred or freak out when you eat too much. Have hope. Go ahead and pull a Scarlett O'Hara: "After all, tomorrow *is* another day."

The great men and women of history have overcome severe problems. That is why they are considered great. History books don't tell of John Doe, who was born to an average family, earned average grades, worked an average job, had an average marriage and average children, and died at an average age. Who cares? It's those who overcame great obstacles and fought great odds that the world wants to remember, to learn of, to be inspired by. So, all you frustrated fatties out there, you have the opportunity to rise above the average, to distinguish yourselves, by overcoming one of the greatest trials that ever beset mankind!

Monday, January 6, 1986
222 pounds

Two and a half months since my last entry. I've dieted for several good spurts during that time. But let's face it, a spurt is a spurt and never results in substantial weight loss. I didn't want to step on the scale this morning, but I forced myself. Oh, horrors! I've gained back almost half of my hard-earned loss. I will not gain any more. I am nearly suicidal. I'm constantly living with that what-am-I-going-to-do-I-can't-stop-eating feeling.

Remember the scene from *Poltergeist* where the jaws of hell envelop the closet doors, sucking everything in? I'm having a similar feeling. It's as if I'm holding on to that door frame with my hands and feet. It would almost be a relief to let myself go and be sucked into that horrible hole, ending it all.

Then again, it's as if I'm being crushed tight into a corner. The pressure of the world—the whole universe, it seems—

keeps smashing me, tighter and tighter. It's sucking up all the air, crushing my lungs, and I can't breathe, and I hurt, and I'm terrified that I won't be able to get another breath, but I'm also terrified to keep on breathing because I'm on my way up the hell scale, and if I gain one more pound, I'll burst or kill myself or something; but I *can't stop* eating, so for sure I *will* gain another pound and—ohhhh! "Please, God, help me!"

I cannot believe that I let myself gain eleven pounds in the past two weeks. Yet I've done it before. When I was pregnant with Matthew, I gained about eighty-five pounds. Uh-huh, you guessed it—I'm pregnant. And while I'm ecstatic at the prospect, I simply cannot gain as I have in the past. I weighed over 270 pounds when I delivered Tiffany. I will not do that to myself again. I cannot; I am now five years older. I might die if I weigh that much.

This pregnancy has kept me continually nauseated, feeling constantly on the verge of throwing up. Whoever named it *morning sickness*? Morning, afternoon, and evening sickness is more like it! I keep thinking that if I could find the right food, my stomach would feel some relief. Nope! All my stomach is feeling is *fatter*!

I keep telling myself that I am eating strictly to make the nausea go away. I know I'm only pretending to myself, but all fat people have worked hard to master that art, the art of deceiving themselves. Pretending it's okay to eat another sandwich because we haven't eaten very much that day, pretending that this is our last—I mean very last—splurge, pretending we can't tell that our clothes are fitting tighter. Why, if we worked that hard at not eating, there would be no more fat people. But we continually pretend, and pretending is such a hard job that we work up quite an appetite.

There is nothing I can eat to make this awful feeling of nausea go away. Time alone will take it away. Two more months, and it should be gone. What am I going to do in the meantime? Gain thirty more pounds? The scary fact is, I could do it. I could easily gain thirty pounds in two months. But I refuse! Even if I have to stay in my room and write twenty-four hours a day to stay away from food. From this second on, there will be no more eating to try to ease the nausea. It never helps. It only makes me fatter. No more eating to try to ease the nausea. It never helps. It only makes me fatter. I'll write it 10,000 times if necessary until it's drilled into my thick skull.

Friday, February 14, 1986
235 pounds

Happy Valentine's Day! Is there anyone more despicable in the entire world than I am? Is there a more pathetic example of womanhood or femininity? Of all His creations, through all the ages, has God been more disappointed in any breathing being than in me? Right now, the answer seems a resounding NO!

My talents and abilities are being wasted on a grand scale. I cannot break out of these carefully handmade chains of despair. The one and only way out is not an escape. It is paying the price. But paying the price—repenting—takes superhuman inner strength. It requires me to completely put heart and soul into His hands . . . but how can I? How can I trust Him when it was He that sent me to this mess?

Dear Heavenly Father,

Can I really write a letter to you and tell you my honest feelings? Will you listen with ears that can hear what words alone cannot express? Will you feel my emotions? Will you agonize over my pain and hurt, and will your breath come in gasps, as mine sometimes does when I feel this is truly the end, and I can't go on another minute? Will you weep with me till your eyes are puffy and swollen and achy as mine?

Oh, Father, this is all part of your plan. You *knew* I would live to this horrible day. You *knew* I would be this miserable, this morbidly obese, this unorganized, this out of control.

How could you send me here? Can't you see that my body is so fat it is causing my soul to suffer the pangs of hell? Even in my imperfections, I love my little ones too much to send them to such a life as this. Even I, with only an earthly capacity for love, would rather see them dead than have them suffer daily misery such as mine. Why did you do this to me, Father? Won't you be merciful and end it all for me?

My earthly father tried, in his own gruff, uneducated way, to love me. But we never talked, I never felt his support in my activities, and seldom felt his arms around me. As a child, I needed that radically, but I need it more today.

Oh, I have felt moments of inexpressible joy. I've gloried over birds and butterflies and babies, but it's like a book I read once . . . long ago. It's an elusive memory. It's not real. Only this present ache is real. Do you know all my thoughts before I write them down? Can you understand me? Do you care about me? Not as a part of humankind, but *me*? I need to know. I need your help. And, if it's not too late, I need your love.

Could you please write back soon and tell me what to do? I can't go on much longer.

> From,
> Rosemary
> I came to Earth on June 18, 1952.
> Remember me?

Sunday, May 18, 1986, 9:20 A.M.
265 pounds

The whole world knows what I've been up to for the last three months! Take a look, one horrifying look. Yes, folks, it's fat ol' me again. Porker city. You know that fifty-four pounds I lost? Well, I found it again. Yup. All fifty-four pounds—with about ten to boot. Gasp! How could I? I ate like a pig—what do you think!?

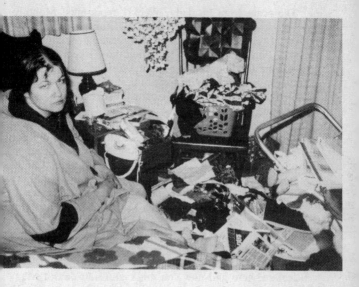

February 1986, 235 pounds. It is no wonder that such depressing thoughts escaped my pen at a time when I was depression personified.

In all fairness, I must give myself a little credit. By the end of May 1985, I'd lost 54 pounds, bringing me down to a paltry 200. I felt almost cute and sexy. Didn't matter that I weighed one-tenth of a ton! Compared to 250, I felt cute and sexy, and this is my diary, so I can write what I want.

I purposely became pregnant around the middle of May, still trying to be careful of what I was eating. When I lost the baby at the end of June, it mentally signaled the immediate end of my glorious diet. I didn't lose another pound after that, but I give myself credit for keeping off most of those rotten fifty pounds for the next six months.

I was thrilled when I became pregnant again. But woe is

me. The scale crept up daily. Weekly freak-outs. Monthly horrors. How could I do it to myself? During the first four months of pregnancy, I was constantly nauseated. I felt as if I had the flu for 120 days. That whole time I kept thinking, "If I eat the right thing, a sandwich, a cracker, some vanilla ice cream, *something* will settle my stomach." Ha! I was almost right. It settled *in* my stomach—and my thighs and my chin and my upper arms.

Then I pulled out all the stops. I ripped them out and threw them away. Those stops were nowhere to be seen! When I was no longer nauseated—and the stops were no longer in existence—look out, we are talking bingeing here. Candy bars nearly every day. Then I discovered a marvelous, new stomach antacid—Mint Love-Its. If you have never eaten a Love-It ice cream bar, you are in for a delight. And *Mint* Love-Its are especially wonderful because everyone knows that mint settles your stomach. Besides, it's the same shape as Rolaids, only 100 times bigger and chocolate-coated. Ah! Such rationalization. Such self-deception.

I declare, here and now, on this eighteenth day of May, in the year of our Lord nineteen hundred and eighty six: I am putting on the brakes. I am coming to a screeching halt. I declare myself officially back on my diet, exercises and all. It doesn't matter that I am six months pregnant. Can't I do a leg lift or swing my arms in a circle? Can't I give up candy, ice cream, and pastry? Does my baby require chocolate to develop normally?

This baby is due in exactly three months, and I will lose no less than thirty pounds. I'll weigh no more than 235 pounds when I deliver this baby. As dreadful as that sounds, it's forty pounds less than the last time I delivered a baby. I'm going to win this war. Before I'm through, every candy bar invented, every chocolate chip created, every ice cream cone scooped up, will surrender. Carrying white flags, they will march before me and bow down and admit that I have won, that I am *their* master, at last!

I just read this entry to Allen. Considering my gross obesity and my pregnant condition, I laughingly asked, "After the way I have described myself, can you think of anything you'd rather do than go to bed with me?'' Allen, with little hesitation: ''Yeah, I'd rather have a Mint Love-It.''

Friday, October 3, 1986
269 pounds

Almost five months since I have written. I have been upset and depressed. I weighed over 300 pounds when Tyler was born on the tenth of August. Of course, one has to take into consideration that I *was* nine months pregnant. That should count for at least 165 extra pounds, right? Brother! What do I think I'm giving birth to, a Mack truck?

Dear baby Tyler weighed nine pounds, fifteen ounces, and

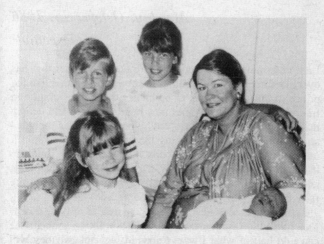

August 10, 1986, 310 pounds. My all-time high, when not pregnant. Here I am, surrounded by Jennifer, Matthew, and Tiffany. Even my beautiful, big, 9-pound, 15-ounce baby Tyler couldn't camouflage that hip!

I lost an astonishing total of ten pounds, one ounce more than he weighed. I was still just as fat, except my stomach felt like well-kneaded bread dough instead of a basketball. But it stuck out almost as far.

A surprised acquaintance asked me the first day of school, "You haven't had that little one yet?" "Well, excuuuuse me!" I wanted to shout. "You haven't had any lessons in etiquette yet?" I was mortified! I wanted to take a peashooter and aim it right at her flat, taut stomach, and then sink into a deep, dark hole. But I knew she was right. I've looked pregnant for fourteen years, since I was three months along with my first child. After my whopping ten-pound weight loss from Tyler's birth, I still weighed an unfathomable 300-plus pounds. Yes, I looked *very* pregnant, but I still hated her for asking.

Monday, October 13, 1986
263 pounds

I am determined to overcome this hideous monster that has overtaken my body. Sometimes I feel a part of me is like the prince in *Sleeping Beauty* as he battles the vicious dragon to free the princess. Remember how huge and ugly and deadly that dragon was? It's crazy, but sometimes it's as though I am also the dragon, terrorizing the prince inside of me! I'll raise my program, my workbook, as my "sword" and see if I can't cut away the dragon—the ugly fat—that surrounds and hides this beautiful princess, the real me! This is one fairy tale that I'm going to make come true.

I really am a sleeping beauty. Except instead of lying down, I've lived the last fourteen years in a walking semi-life. I can't do half of what I want to do. My fat not only disables me, it inhibits me. Many things I physically *can't* do, and others I'm too embarrassed to do. It's a lose-lose situation. Well, look out, world—I'm going to start lose-losing!

No one knows I'm changing, but I am! I want to be better,

inside and out. I am happy to report that as I improve the outside of me, the inside is pulled along by osmosis.

This seven pounds has disappeared slowly. It was an emotional challenge to diet so faithfully and lose only two pounds in the first eleven days. But, as will always happen to the faithful dieter, I eventually experienced a significant weight loss. In two weeks, I lost seven pounds. That's fourteen pounds a month. I can't give up. "Day-by-day" can be frustrating, even depressing. But when I look at the whole picture, a month at a time, I can and will lose weight. So can everyone else!

Beware of the person who says, "I dieted faithfully and didn't lose a pound." Come on, be honest, how long were you *on* the diet? Ten minutes? Oh, please! Don't try to kid *me*. I'm fat, too. I know all the secrets. The diet worked fine; you chose not to work the diet—not long enough, anyway. You were probably snacking or sneaking or cramming or bingeing much of the time. Let me put it this way: Don't trust that person with your child's trick-or-treat candy.

Tuesday, October 14, 1986
263 pounds

I watched the movie *The Miracle Worker* last night. I had seen it several times before, but the repeat impact is always as awe-inspiring as the first. Helen Keller's world was totally void of reason. She stumbled along in the dark, both physically and mentally. The instant when Helen realized that there was meaning to life, a reason for her existence, a way to communicate, was one of the most moving moments of all time.

I try to live with her through her sudden burst into the world of words. It was more dramatic than if she were suddenly to see. In a small way, I know how Helen Keller felt. To a tiny degree, I've experienced her revelation. I know how it feels to be totally without hope. I know how it feels to be locked

away in a dark and miserable world where no one understands
me, where I don't understand myself, where I don't even like
myself.

But thanks to God alone, I also know how it feels to exult
in that awe-inspiring moment when a person realizes the sun
does shine, the world *is* wonderful, that one *can* become a
whole person again.

Thursday, October 30, 1986
259 pounds

If you can say "the day before Halloween" and not feel
elated and stop-dead-in-your-tracks terrified at the same time
. . . you are blessed indeed. For that means you have never
been fat. That means you've never known the delightful anticipation of all the yummy morsels about to march into your
life, right there in plain sight, in the deceptive form of your
children's Halloween candy. Oh, but all you *fatties* know.
You'll lie in bed at night, envisioning those chocolate delights
till you can no longer resist—and you'll have to run in and
sneak (steal) a few bars from each child's hoard.

Here's the kicker. They are such convenient little bars,
specially packaged for the big night. Surely they can't hurt
you. Why, they are only one or two bites at the most! So
you rationalize, as you down ten bars.

Friday, October 31, 1986
260 pounds

So the evil day has arrived. I still have not purchased any
candy for the soon-to-be-arriving trick-or-treaters. No, that
is not quite true. I *had* purchased my trick-or-treat candy.
But—okay, there is simply no other way to say it—I ate it.

I was at the store last Saturday. I'd been faithful to my
diet all day. Then I foolishly bought a one-pound bag each

of Baby Ruths and Butterfingers. I knew from the first moment that I was going to eat a few bars. Oh, I *told* myself I absolutely would not *touch* that candy. Yet, deep down, I knew I was doomed. I knew better than to buy it, even though it was on sale.

Later, my sister Debbie said, "Ya' dummy! Whatcha go and buy the best stuff for? Of course, you'll eat it, ya' nut! Don't you know you're supposed to buy the nonchocolate stuff, so you won't be tempted?"

My surface thoughts had been so noble: "I'll get Baby Ruths and Butterfingers because they were my favorites when I went trick-or-treating as a child." But my deep-down thoughts were a little more honest: "I'm dying for a Baby Ruth!"

When I stood at the checkout stand, I didn't have to feel sick to my stomach with the shame of being a big ol' fatso buying candy again. You see, that's one fabulous blessing of Halloween. Fat people can buy bags and *bags* of candy because it's all for the dear little trick-or-treaters, right? HA! I'm sure!

The clerk at the cash register almost did me in. Here's an exact quote from that lanky little wench: "Oh, I don't know how you people have the willpower to buy your Halloween candy early. Why, I'd just *have* to eat it!" Oh, not me, thin cheeks. Why, I wouldn't dream of it. The thought never crossed my mind. I almost wished one of her skinny, bony fingers would get pinched in the cash register drawer.

I offered a rather sick smile as a reply to her ignorant, typical thin-person words. The real irony of the situation was this: I was praying that the person in line behind me hadn't heard the clerk's remark about willpower, while at the same time, I was scheming the quickest way to get one of those chocolate-coated devils past my lips. I could hardly control the urge long enough to get out of her eyesight.

The second I knew I was safe, I reached into the sack as discreetly as possible. I tore open the plastic bag and grasped a Baby Ruth. Ah, I could almost taste it. At this point, I was nearly trembling for chocolate. I ripped off the wrapper and plunked the whole thing in my mouth. Now I could calm down. Now I could relax. Now I could eat a Butterfinger.

I strolled through the grocery section, steadily munching away. Surely, no one noticed me eating—I was so cautious, so careful. (Oh, please! Who am I kidding? I weigh over 250 pounds! Right there you know I didn't have a chance to escape attention. *Everyone* notices fat people.) I'm sure each time I ripped open another wrapper, someone heard it! I was acutely ashamed of my behavior, humiliated at my own lack of self-control, but I went right on eating like a crazy lady. Yup, folks, I ate the whole pound of Baby Ruths and over half the Butterfingers that same night.

And what was my very first thought upon waking the next morning? "Oh, glory be! There are Butterfingers left!" I cautiously slipped out of bed. Moving quietly, I retrieved that bag of Butterfingers from its hiding place. Taking great pains not to let the plastic bag rustle, I sneaked out of our room and down the hall. Thank goodness Allen is such a deep sleeper. Ahhhh! What could be better than an early Sunday morning to myself? What could be better? Exactly what I had: an early Sunday morning to share with a half pound of Butterfingers.

At this point, let me take a moment to expound on this particular bag of Butterfingers. These bars were not regular size or snack size or—heaven forbid!—giant size. No, the clever makers of these yummy little morsels dubbed them "fun size." *Fun Size?* Oh, I get it! You get to a really fun size if you eat them. Fun size—it just kills me. I tell you, the more I eat, the funner life gets!

One by one, I ate those incredibly fun little Butterfingers. One by one, they disappeared down my throat, only to reappear on my stomach, hips, shoulders, chin, and cheeks. (Oh, fun, fun, fun!) Finally, there were only seven left. Perfect. I'd use three for my children's lunches and four as treats for the children I baby-sit. *Suuuure* I would. "Six little, five little, four little candy bars—three little candy bars left." Well, At least *my* three children would each have one in their lunches. *Suuuure* they would. I was able to rationalize eating

Matthew's because at that time he was trying to drop a couple of pounds (two bars left). And Jeremy was currently having a love affair with Clearasil (one left). Oh, surely there was *some* reason Jennifer didn't deserve one (none left).

Whew! Actually, I'm glad I ate them all because now I don't have to worry about them anymore. Oh, what a poor little fool I am. I know only too well that "now" is when I really have to start worrying about them—now, when they have become a permanent part of me!

Friday, November 7, 1986
258 pounds

I am furious with you, Debbie. *Sure* this is a great idea, this "do your checklist or do my housework!" agreement. It's 12:28 A.M., and here I am writing in this dumb diary because I didn't do it earlier today. If I don't write today, I'll have to work at your house, Debbie. I guess the plan is working because I sure wouldn't have done any of the things on this list if I didn't have to clean your house for *not* doing them. So I'm writing. So try to make me clean your house! So there.

Today we viewed the family portraits we recently had taken. Oh, horrors. I am ugliness personified. I am so fat. My cheeks could be filled with helium and lift a car. It is so revealing to look at my own fat self. It is a miserable experience. Surely I'm not that *fat* person staring back at me. I look like Moby Dick. Everyone says the picture looks good, just like me—beautiful. Oh, I hate them all. Do you hear me? *I hate you all!* I *don't* look like that. This is only a mask. I can hardly wait till the unveiling. The photos are slightly out of focus. Wish I could blame the photographer for my blubber as well as the blur.

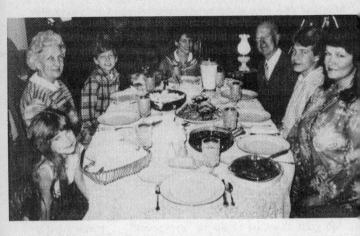

November 1986, 258 pounds. Thanksgiving dinner with Allen's parents and my children. I'm thankful I no longer have to sit in that hideous, unfeminine, typical-obese-lady sitting position!

Sunday, November 23, 1986
252 pounds

I cannot believe how difficult it is to do something that is supremely important and that I want desperately. It seems as though big rocks are being dumped in my path at every turn. Every day that I do my checklist, I am faithful to my diet, and every day I don't do my list, I am terrible on my diet. I try to get away with *mentally* checking it off each day, but it isn't the same. There is no substitute for "getting the lead out" and putting it down in writing.

I have an intense desire to be thin. I want pretty clothes. Last night I enjoyed Christmas shopping with my husband. It's fun to buy clothes for the children, but *I* want to dress nicely, too. I want to feel "stylish." I want a little variety in my clothes. Variety—schmariety! I want to be warm this winter.

It's horribly hard to lay out the money for a warm coat. A coat that fits me. A coat I can button up. I keep telling myself, "I will buy a new coat when I lose some weight." The thought of spending one hundred dollars or more for a size-twenty-four anything is unthinkable. Furthermore, trying on those huge tents is emotionally devastating, so I stick with the coat I've outgrown. Those miserable six inches down the front of me are exposed to the freezing weather because I'm too fat to button my coat.

A few moments ago, Allen made me furious with one of his famous, dumb comments. I was just getting ready to lambast him with the written word! I was going to make this page burn. But drats! He came in and apologized before I put pen to paper. Now all the anger and venom have dissipated, so I won't be able to do my original feelings justice. But I will give it a good try:

I was writing in my diary when Allen came upstairs. I called out to him, my dear little voice filled with pride and enthusiasm: "I'm writing in my diary, and I've already done my exercises!" (Could anyone be more charming, clever, or devoted to a diet than I?) His immediate response? In a rather know-it-all, better-than-thou voice: "On Sunday?" Oh, the dirty rat! Oh, the stinking bum! Sure, Allen! Fourteen years of being a tub o' lard. Fourteen years of tears, self-hatred, and agonizing failure. Fourteen years of breaking every food-related health law on the books—and you give me an "On Sunday?" Oh, please. I know we try to "keep the Sabbath Day holy," but could God possibly mind if—in the privacy of my own home—I touched my toes and reached up a few times? We're not talking health spa here or jogging down the highway. We're not talking swimming, biking, or horseback riding. I did a few simple exercises on my front room floor, for crying out loud. I need the motivation. I need the upper I feel when I'm all done, and probably more than anything else, I need your support!

Tuesday, January 6, 1987
255 pounds

Nineteen eighty-seven. The sweet sound of success. The year of happiness. The year of new beginnings. The year for *me*. *My* year! This is the year I change. I mean rip-snortin' change here. I mean real, dig-it-out-by-the-roots-and-burn-the-blasted-habit change. This year I will lose over 100 pounds. This year I will clean my house. No, I mean *clean* my house. I don't mean stuff-all-the-junk-in-a-box-and-hide-it clean. I mean every box sorted out, every dresser drawer straightened, every closet organized. I mean every window glistening, every carpet shampooed, every cupboard door with a nonstick surface. I mean every switch plate defingermarked, every cobweb removed, every door frame dusted! *I mean clean!*

This year I will emerge from this horrid imitation of a humanoid, and the real me—the thin, sweet, organized me—will appear. Only the name will remain the same. All else changes. Well, except maybe my eyebrows. I do have nice eyebrows. And I like the color of my eyes. But my cheeks look like the never-ending story. I'd like to lose about one half of each. Even my nose looks rather fat. Yet, in spite of my fat nose, I'm excited. Okay. Don't laugh. I have to say it: "This is it. I really mean it!"

Thursday, January 8, 1987
255 pounds

Hallelujah! I get to do my exercises! Do you detect a little sarcasm here? How wrong you are. There is not a little sarcasm—there is a great deal of sarcasm. I need to exercise, for eventually it will help me. But right now, the thought of exercising repulses me! I don't want to lift one leg. I don't want to touch one toe. I want to lie here and watch TV forever!

Monday, January 12, 1987
255 pounds

I'm souped up. (Wouldn't you know it, a food adjective!) The joy of accomplishment is splendid. I can hardly stand the sweet taste of success. Eureka! That's it. I have to get the sweet taste of chocolate out of my mouth, so the sweeter taste of success can come in! I like that thought.

I weighed a disgusting 255 this morning. Since I feel like I'm in the jaws of hell, I wish they'd chew me up for a while and keep the devilish, ugly fat me and spew out the beautiful inner core—the real me, the thin, sweet, successful me! I'm going to win this war! The battles have been many, the losses devastating, but victory is just around the corner. I must get to sleep. Because I'm doing my checklist, I can look forward to awaking with hope in my heart. What a change from a few days ago!

Wednesday, January 14, 1987, 10:00 A.M.
255 pounds

Suuuure I'll stick to my diet. Oh, life is hell. I mean it. Life *is* hell! I hate it. I detest waking up each morning. More of the same. Misery. Agony. Torture. Disappointment. Lack of sleep. Lack of love. Shame. Dirty dishes. Overeating. Yelling at children. Messy rooms. Junk, junk, junk! No one trying. No one caring. Baby crying. Meals to cook. Doorbell ringing—all day. Baby-sitting kids, running and screaming indoors. Why get up? If I slept all day, the house couldn't get any messier. I never get anything accomplished anyway. Everything is partway done. Allen tried to help me, but we're talking *Mission Impossible* here.

Good grief! There is not a clean spoon in my kitchen. Every diaper in this house is dirty. My bed hasn't been changed for over a month. I haven't washed my windows for years. My toilets have brown rings. My garage is a death trap. My attic is crammed full of junk. My Christmas tree is half undecorated. My "writing desk" is stacked two feet high with papers to sort and file. I weigh over 250 pounds, making it difficult to bend over. I have to kick things out of the way as I walk down the hall. I have to climb in on Allen's side of the bed at night because of all the junk piled on the floor on my side. Half my children wet their beds. I baby-sit seven kids a day. I am over $50,000 in debt. I'm in a state of severe depression. I am contemplating suicide.

Somehow, it doesn't make sense. Somehow, it wasn't supposed to be like this. Somehow, I wanted more. A ray of hope once in a while. One day of my children getting their responsibilities done on their own. One day of a clean house. One hour of a thin body. One full night's sleep. One night of not worrying about bills. One day of not losing control, not screaming at the children or Allen. Just one day. Dear God, would one day be so hard for you to let go of?

I can't kill myself. It would be a dirty trick. To leave and never look back wouldn't be fair, either. It sounds so sweet. But even Looney Tunes, tub-o'-lard me can see the injustice. Poor Allen. If I killed myself, he'd have to arrange for the funeral. He can't afford it. And either escape—death or leaving—would leave the poor man devastated. Oh, don't get me wrong. I don't flatter myself. He'd be better off without me, but if I feel lost in this mountain of a mess we supposedly call home, he would drown. If he were suddenly solely responsible for this eighteen-room-plus-attic-plus-garage junk box, he'd keel over then and there. Then I'd be responsible for murder, too, and Allen's life is worth something. At least, it could have been, but it's sure gone downhill since he met me. He has to spend at least half of his time wondering when I'm going to explode next, and the other half wondering in which direction my wrath will flow. He has to ask daily for a clean shirt, clean socks, clean underwear, or clean hanky. He never knows if there will be a dinner ready when he gets home. His only escape from the mess, the total chaos, is going to work.

How did I ever get into this mess? One little paper, one

dropped article of clothing, one misplaced item, one un-
washed dish at a time. But can it ever be reversed? It took
me fifteen years to reach this state of chaos. Can I wait fifteen
more years to undo all of the mess I've made? Poor Allen.
I feel so sorry for him. If he had never met me, he could
have married a woman who would have lived up to the ideal
I had hoped to be for him. She could have raised his children
better. Anyone could improve on what I've done. There is
one thing in my favor. No one could have given him more
beautiful children. I do find joy in that. Ironically, it's the
one thing I had nothing to do with. Let's face it, looks are
sheer heredity and luck!

1:15 P.M. Talked with Debbie for one hour. One silly little
hour, and I feel much better, more confident, more hopeful.

Wednesday, January 21, 1987
255 pounds

I want skinniness more than anything right now. More than
a million dollars. More than good health. More than perfect
children. Heck, even more than sex! After all, everything
would be better if I were thin. So what am I doing? At least
this morning I am sincerely trying. I started at the top and
worked straight down my Daily Checklist. I need it. Some
semblance of order. Some rhyme or reason.

The very first thing on my checklist is prayer. I need God's
help to overcome this addiction. I am desperate for that certain
inner strength that can come only from Him. I have not been
diligent in saying my daily prayers. If I have to stay on my
knees all day to keep myself out of the kitchen, I'll do it. I
like the saying: If you're not communicating with God, it's
not He who hung up the phone.

Dreaming of being thin helps me to stick to my diet. One
of my dreams is to be thin enough to deliver a surprise birthday pizza to Jeremy at school. I want him to be glad, not
crestfallen, to see me coming. By September 23, Jeremy's

birthday, I should weigh 155 pounds—*or less!* I look pretty good at 155. I will deck myself out like a model straight off the cover of a high-fashion magazine! Considering my present weight, that's some fancy dream. Yes, for me, it would be as grand as a trip to Europe. To have my Jeremy proud to have me visit him at school. "Yeah, guys—this is my mom!" How tragic that my fat has prevented me from doing countless fun, nice, crazy things for my husband and children.

I'm hungry. I'm feeling real, legitimate, stomach-growling hunger here. What melodious sounds. I must march into the kitchen, eat only what's on my list, and not go berserk. There is a batch of cookie dough in there. A living, breathing monster, waiting to grab my hand and force its way into my mouth.

Saturday, January 24, 1987
253 pounds

I was deeply discouraged a couple of days ago. I hadn't even stepped out of bed, and already everything seemed wrong. I asked Allen, "Why should I even *try* to diet?" His answer was so simple: "Because it's the only problem in your world you have complete control over." It was a resoundingly true statement. Today I will use that control to my advantage. No one forces me down on the floor, ties my hands behind my back, and shoves food in my mouth. No one chains me up and makes me eat till I'm sick. No one puts giant magnets in my car, causing it to pull over at every corner store so I can buy a candy bar, or to Arby's so I can chomp on a chocolate chip cookie or two . . . or six. (Have you ever tasted an Arby's chocolate chip cookie? Mmmmm. They are good. Oh, good, schmood; they are scrumptious, they are divine, they are . . . no, stop! Get a grip, Rosemary! Sure, Arby's chocolate chip cookies are good, but a size ten is better!)

Sunday, January 25, 1987
253 pounds

In reading some of the poignantly sad entries of the past few months, I am ashamed. Yet those have been, and still often are, my true feelings. I could write all sorts of happy and beautiful lies, but I think of Shakespeare's words, "To thine own self, be true." My diary will be worthless to me if I am not honest with myself. Today I must write about something that fills my soul with hope and joy and love:

THE OTHER MAN
by Rosemary Green

I love my husband very much—
 I've been fifteen years his wife.
So it surprises even me to find a
 new man in my life.
I suppose I saw it coming,
 but I had no self-control!
He hypnotized away my heart;
 he mesmerized my soul.

He never *said* he loved me,
 we'd no need to verbalize.
His charming smile said enough
 . . . and that look—deep in his eyes.
Oh, he's made my life just crazy,
 but I cannot let him go!
I think about him day and night;
 I really love him so.
My husband knows about us.
 He thinks it rather fun
That I should love this guy so much
 . . . my precious, newborn son!

I feel almost worshipful of my precious Jon Tyler. For these past five months, he has brought sunshine into my bleakest day, my darkest hour. My love for him is immeasurable. I am overwhelmingly grateful for the precious gift of motherhood. There is no experience on earth that can compare to the delight and sacred reverence one feels when holding a baby.

Tuesday, March 31, 1987
262 pounds

I am depressed. I'm so miserable and humiliated over my appearance that I hate to go to church, let alone out to dinner. It's hard to comprehend this much misery. I am so morbidly obese that when I sit down, this huge, massive bulk is between my lap and my bosom. It's called a stomach.

I remember a song from my childhood: "So high, you can't go over it. So low, you can't go under it. So wide, you can't go around it . . . ya gotta go through that door." I've found myself mumbling these horrible words to that tune lately: "I'm so fat, I can't hide it. So huge, I can't get away from it. So wide, I can't move around much . . . I gotta go lose some weight!"

Elizabeth Taylor is gorgeous again. I saw her last night on a Barbara Walters special. She's down to a size five, a dramatic drop from the obese woman she had become. She is an inspiration. After viewing her "before" and "after" pictures last night, I felt determined to try one more time. But I'm afraid to get too excited for myself. I can't take many more failures. Just writing in my diary stimulates the deeply buried emotion of pride that comes from triumph over self. I am apprehensive as I begin to nibble at the sweet taste of success again.

Thursday, April 2, 1987
260 pounds

Being fat is a handicap, as real as being blind, deaf, or crippled. The ugly difference is that we fat people live constantly with the hideous knowledge that it's *our fault*. Worse yet, we know we could correct it. We can literally "eat ourselves well." No blind person can do that. As a result, we live in a horrid, know-we-can-fix-it-but-not-doing-anything-about-it existence, somewhere between a hope for a better future and a miserable now.

I feel like the character Robert Frost writes of in his immortal poem, "The Road Not Taken." I also have two roads before me. One is the well-worn road of obesity. Eat, eat, eat. Show no self-control, no discipline. Just look at the millions of fat feet traveling it daily. That road is an eight-lane, fully paved highway.

But today, I will repeat Frost's line, "And I? I took the one less traveled by." The unmarked road. The vague path, with bushes encroaching and weeds springing up in the middle, but still, the road that leads to a thinner me, a happier life. My weight alone is enough to make deep ruts in this unmarked road, so, hopefully, it will be easier for others to follow.

My muscles are sore this morning from extensive exercise yesterday. Isn't that wonderful? I ache all over. Isn't that grand? As soon as I am through writing, I will do my exercises for today. In a few days, the aches will be gone, and I'll feel like Jane Fonda. (Okay, so it might take me a few weeks to feel like Jane!)

Last night Allen took me out to dinner. I fooled myself into thinking I could handle an all-you-can-eat salad bar. Who am I kidding? "All-I-can-eat" is *never* a diet meal. I ate enough to last a week! When I was completely stuffed, I shoveled in some chocolate pudding. Feeling horribly guilty over the outrageous amount I had just consumed, I committed to Allen (but over my already empty plate), "I never want to come here again! It's too hard to come to an all-you-can-eat place and eat only what I should.''

I must work to get this if-it's-all-you-can-eat-then-I-have-to-eat-a-ton-to-get-my-money's-worth syndrome out of my head. I must replace it with my own motto: The less I eat, the more I lose.

Wednesday, April 22, 1987
262 pounds

Twenty days since an entry. I faithfully did my Daily Checklist for seven days. Allen commented on how nice it was to see me up, to see me happy. Then I fell off the wagon. Ha! To say "fell off the wagon" is like saying the Elephant Man had a slight puffiness under the eyes! I crashed off the wagon with all the sheer, raw energy of an atom bomb. I ate everything in sight . . . and out of sight. I thought of nothing but food: when I could eat it, where I could buy it, how I could make it, did I have the ingredients to make it? Eat, eat, eat. It's hard work to maintain this physique! And this at a time when we're flat broke! I can't afford ground beef for a casserole, but somehow I always seem to have a dollar for a few sweets.

Am I finally brave enough to write about my sister Rebecca today? I don't know. I do know that I don't *want* to write about her. In fact, it will take extraordinary courage to do so. Okay, I'll blurt it out: I hate Rebecca right now. She's done the dirty deed; she's committed the unpardonable sin. She has lost all her excess weight. She's *skinny*, okay? And I hate her for it! And I hate myself for hating her. But I can't help it. And I'm not going to lie about it.

It's the curse of all fat people. We thoroughly *dislike* skinny people. You know, those waspish-waisted, thin-necked, firm-thighed vixens. The oh-I-better-not-have-dessert-give-me-a-diet-pop, 110-pound glamour girls. Oh, yes, we thoroughly *dislike* them. But give us a fatty that does it, that finally gets thin, that breaks the bonds of hell, and we feel *hatred*. I mean venom. Whenever we're around the ex-lardo, we smile and try to act normal, but inside, undetected, our eyes narrow and send out arrow showers of hatred, of jealousy, of the desire for revenge. It's as if this person attacked us by losing weight, which, in a way, she did. This ex-fatty is now a light to the world: "See, you can do it. I did it. Why don't you just put down the food?" Oh, yes, I feel a real hatred for Rebecca. She is a vivid reminder of my own failure.

I hate every fat-free pound of her. I hate the way she polishes her nails. I hate the way she plucks her eyebrows. I hate the way she crosses her sexy legs. I hate the way she tosses her exotic red hair every time she runs a brush through it. I hate each new size-five outfit she buys. I've gained several pounds just trying to drown out my guilt for feeling hateful!

To be fair to myself, there's a part of me that is also thrilled for Rebecca. She weighs 117 pounds. We're talking high-school weight here. She's gorgeous. She is wearing darling, stylish clothes. Her every step is almost a dance. It's inspiring to look at her and think, "She did it. She escaped. She is beautiful again!" But I cannot deny the hatred I feel.

Oh, God, please help me this one day. I, too, need to be thin again. I've been so depressed, so hard to live with. Help me not to think of food every second today.

When I woke this morning, my first thought was, "What is there to eat? I hope one of the baby-sitting kids brought a treat to share!" Can you believe that? Those thoughts from a grown-up woman who is practically suicidal in her desperation to lose weight. I want to be thin more than anything because losing weight is everything. It's hope, it's fun with my children, it's being able to serve my family, my church, and my fellowmen. It's better mobility, better attitude, better love life. It's everything. *Everything!* Yet my first thought this morning was, "What is there to eat?"

September 26, 1991. That was over four years ago.
I am happy to write that in those four years I have

lost over 70 pounds, and I no longer hate Rebecca.
I'm afraid she found every last pound she lost. And
do you want my honest feeling? It's ugly, but a part
of me is happy. Almost vindictively so. For the first
time in my life, she is much heavier than I am.

  My dream is to reach 125 pounds . . . and I
would love it if Rebecca didn't lose a pound in the
meantime. Oh, I hope she gets skinny and gorgeous
again someday . . . but not till I'm incredibly thin.

Monday, April 27, 1987
262 pounds

Had a sweet talk with my in-laws yesterday. It's nice to know that they love me—fat or thin—but I remember how Allen's father used to show me off to his friends. He was even more proud of me than he was of his prized, purebred Arabian horses. I'm afraid I became "unshowoffable" about 100 pounds ago. No, I don't think he loves me any less, but no one would be excited to show off an original painting—even by Michelangelo—if it were covered with 100 coats of black paint. Okay, give me eight months. I'll look 100 percent different, hopefully 100 pounds different!

I redid my Weight-Loss Goal Calendar today. Funny coincidence. I will reach my goal of 125 on June 18, 1988. My thirty-sixth birthday. Fine! It will be the perfect time to get pregnant. And *voilà*! Another diary: *Nine Months to a Better Me!* I do have this fantasy of being nine months pregnant and looking like something less than Moby Dick. A little watermelon tummy on a thin lady looks so cute. Once in my life, I would like to experience being pregnant and cute!

Saturday, May 2, 1987
255 pounds

I've been depressed for a long time. I even find it hard to go
to church because I am shamed by my own appearance. Still,
sitting next to Allen on Sunday, with the children around us,
is one of the high points of my week. Last Sunday, following
my women's auxiliary meeting, I walked into the chapel for
worship service. As soon as I sat down, I noticed that Allen
was up front in the clerk's seat to take minutes. Yikes! I
thought I would forget how to breathe, I was so upset. I knew
that whoever was asked to be clerk was expected to sit up
there through the whole meeting. That meant that I . . . would
have to sit . . . all by myself. Me and my fat stomach; me
and this other blimp of a person who inhabits my body. Oh,
how dare Allen desert me without letting me know? How
dare he make me sit through an hour and ten minutes of hell?

It had taken all the courage I possessed to make that walk
down the aisle to sit by my children. I felt that every eye in
the chapel was fixed on me. I felt that every head was filled
with the same thoughts as I moved my ''incredible hulk,''
inch by inch, down that long aisle. I could feel their disgust
as they stared at the rolls of fat surrounding my waist. I knew
they were all appalled by the ham-hock size of my upper
arms. I knew they all grimaced at my double chin. I was sure
they could all hear the rough scratching of my nylons as
my thighs rubbed together with each step. I knew they all
wondered, ''What in the world does that woman eat all day
to look like such a balloon?'' I prayed that by holding the
baby, I could camouflage the fact that my arms can't rest
comfortably on my sides because of the humongous amount
of flab on each hip and fat under each arm.

Those horrible feelings of paranoia about my obesity were
making it difficult to breathe evenly. Then I realized that
Allen, my crutch, my link with normalcy, my she-must-give-
some - worthwhile - contribution - to - the - human - race - if - *he* -
is-with-her message was not going to be with me. I became

frantic. I had to repeat, "Calm down, think for a moment, don't stand up and scream. Take a deep breath."

I thought, "Okay. What shall I do? I'll leave. I'll just get up and walk . . . and walk . . . and walk down that long aisle—again? Oh, no, not that. I'd faint. My knees would give out before I reached the door. To have to experience that horrible scrutiny again—head-on—no, never that! So I'll sit here. I'll try to squeeze myself into a smaller space. I'll try to disappear. I'll try to die. I think I *am* dying. I'll concentrate on holding in my stomach, scrunching my shoulders together, tucking up my chin, and keeping my knees together. An hour and ten minutes. Oh, Allen, how could you ever do this to me?"

Needless to say, after the meeting, when Allen came down from his perch to ask about dinnertime, my first comment was, "If you ever do that to me again without warning me, I'll leave!" Perhaps if he'd understood my deep distress, he'd have been sweet and understanding. I can't remember his response as he abruptly turned and walked away, but it was the final push I needed to go over the edge that day. I was so angry with him. When I arrived home from church, I marched right in and ate four maple bars. I was going to "show Allen good" this time, but all I did was make one more roll on myself to suck in, tuck up, scrunch together, or try to hide.

It was a miserable Sabbath. But somehow, I have been able to "click" on to my diet again, and I've lost seven pounds in the last five days. I feel hopeful.

Last night was Friday, our "date" night. Allen played drums at a wedding reception and didn't get home till 10:00. He opened the paper to see what was on TV, then continued to read. I wasn't mad at the time. After I mentioned we might do something more exciting than watch TV, I continued to work on my checklist. In a few moments I asked him, "Do you want to see something inspiring?"

"Yes," he answered. I showed him the progress I was making toward my weight-loss goals. He said it was neat that I was ahead of schedule. But he soon showed his true colors, his lack of genuine interest. I proudly turned to the new chart I had made that day. But he didn't look; he kept getting ready for bed. Then he asked something about how much longer I needed to talk to him, because he wanted to watch a documentary that was starting on TV. This, on my "date" night. My one night a week to have him all to myself. This, after fourteen years of my being 100-plus pounds overweight. This, after five days of success I needed to share. This, after countless hours through the years of seeing me weep uncontrollably over my obesity. This, from a man who has to make love to a tub-o'-lard butterball. A television program was more important than I was!

I held my temper. Oh, the words that sprang, unbidden, to my mind and almost to my lips. I was deeply hurt. I slammed my workbook shut, wanting to let Allen know I had just closed him out of my world. I slammed my book, but I held my temper. Allen ended up yelling at me, "You make me sick. You're uneducated. You can't appreciate any kind of documentary film because you don't want to learn anything."

Liar! It was I who had wanted to watch *Shoah* the last four nights in a row. And it was 100 percent documentary. Liar. I didn't say it, but I can *look* pretty wicked when I want to.

Sigh . . . what did I want? How would I have liked Allen to respond last night? What did I need? Okay, I am Sick, with a capital *S*. I'm horrible to live with and hideous to look at! But I'm trying to change. I'm on my diet right now; I'm high. But I need support to keep me there! (Even if only once a week—on my date night.) I would have liked him to sit down on the bed for a few minutes, to stop getting ready for bed, or to say, "Let me finish getting into my pajamas, so I'll be more comfortable." I would have liked him to ignore the TV. To act interested in my success. To show he cared.

After he said his mean words that cut me to the quick (and, believe me, with all this fat to protect me, my quick is hard to find), I didn't respond. I held back the venom. Maybe that's not so good either because that meant the venom stayed inside of me. I looked at him for a long time while he watched his precious TV program. I hated him. I pitied him, the fool. There is a great deal of me locked away inside this fat shell that he doesn't know. He has no idea of what I have to offer him, to us, to our family. I thought, "I will get thin. I will get thin, and then I will leave him. I will be free then. I will have a choice then. I will be able to walk down an aisle and hold my head high because I won't have to concentrate on holding my stomach in."

It turned out to be an excellent program. (Allen is quite selective in the few TV programs he watches.) It was the story of Mendel and how he became known as "the father of genetics." He was not acknowledged for his brilliant success until after his death. The end of the program was heart-rending. An extremely foolish and prejudiced man took Mendel's place as abbot of the monastery. He burned all Mendel's journals and the records of his experiments. I was appalled as his books were thrown on the fire. I wanted to scream, "No, no, no, they're precious. They're important. Don't burn them. Oh, you fools." I wanted to jump up and pull them from the fire. Then it hit me. That was exactly the way Allen made me feel tonight. He pushed me into the fire, not with his hands, but with his cruel, barbed words, with his lack of support for my "experiment," with his lack of interest in my life. I pray the damage is not irreparable.

I need to quit thinking about that experience. I will write about Emily. I'm sick for her. It's painful to think about her. Emily had been dangerously overweight for years. She was the quintessential example of a roly-poly butterball! Then, about two years ago, she started on a doctor-supervised liquid diet, and she did it; she lost over 100 pounds. She became *thin*. She looked fabulous! Emily was wearing tuck-in blouses and belts and looking the epitome of chic.

She had reached her goal. She stopped the liquid diet. She stopped any diet. After that long struggle, she's probably sixty pounds overweight again. Oh, the poor woman. While eating a candy bar two days ago, she lamented to me, "Oh, to be thin again!"

Even her dearest friends daren't say anything to Emily.

It's gone too far to mention. We all pretend she is still a size nine and try not to stare at her as she eats any and every thing in sight. Only a few months ago we were bragging her up like crazy. Every few minutes someone called her skinny or sexy or told her she looked like a model. Now what do we do? Is someone going to march up to her and say, "Hey, you look fat. What did you do, gain sixty pounds?" That is not a healthy question!

If you're one of the "Big Is Beautiful" brainwashers out there, I ask you point-blank: If big is so beautiful, why haven't I been complimented one single time in the last nineteen years about how terrific I look as an extremely obese person? Not *once* has anyone said, "Hey, you must have gained twenty pounds since I last saw you . . . you look great!" Not once. But *every* time I lose twenty-five or more pounds, people shower me with compliments. They want to know how I'm doing it. *Every* time. "Big Is Beautiful"? I think not!

This entry needs a funny story. Yesterday, I called my sister Debbie and told her I'd lost another pound. She was happy for me. "So how are *you* doing?" I asked.

"Oh, I fluctuated up two pounds. I'm not really up, I just fluctuated." Pause.

Me: "Debbie, do you know how dumb you sound? You didn't fluctuate. You *gained* two pounds!"

Debbie: "Dang it!" Well, that's the story of Debbie's fluctuation. Fluctuation and rationalization. Two words for me to stay away from!

And here's something else to stay away from: drive-through restaurants! Yesterday, I was stopped at a light, minding my own business, when I saw this humongous man pulling into a drive-through line. When I say humongous, I mean it. I had to do a double take just to take him all in. He had no neck. Disgusting, puffed skin fell from his chin to his chest. One huge elbow was resting outside of the window. There are no words to describe satisfactorily his size *or* the pity I felt for him.

He'll never know what a favor he did me! He kept me

from that very drive-through line. I saw shades of myself—
a little farther down the road of life, perhaps, for I'm not that
fat yet, but I am well on my way. I'd have died before pulling
in behind him. But the instant before I saw him, I was already
thinking, "Hmmmm . . . do I have a dollar in my purse?
What could I get for a dollar at Taco Time?"

Monday, May 11, 1987
249 pounds

Yes, folks, that's one seldom-mentioned sin of our society:
drive-through restaurants. Besides wasting a bazillion gallons
of gas a day and polluting the atmosphere, they are a significant health threat to fat people.

A great percentage of cars in the drive-through lines are
driven by the obese. Most of the time, we fatties don't have
the nerve or energy to haul ourselves out of our cars, plop
up to the counter, and order. We feel hidden and protected
in our little cubbyholes. And if we order enough for four,
surely the cashier will think it's for others at home. We pray
she won't notice our double chin or our Sumo-size upper
arm.

That reminds me of a story my friend Melissa told me.
Before the day of the drive-through, Melissa would go into
a fast-food restaurant and order two burgers and two fries—
for herself, a snack on the way home from school. (Can you
believe it? All that for a snack!) Melissa would have died if
the cashier thought it was all for her, so she would also order
two drinks. Melissa was sure the cashier would automatically
assume there was another person outside in the car. Surely
no one would order two drinks for herself. The pathetic part
of this story is that Melissa was more concerned about the
opinion of the cashier, a total stranger, than she was about
her own health and appearance.

Saturday, May 30, 1987
247 pounds

Now here is a funny experience. I shall title it: ''Thinking Thin at the Dentist's Office.''

I have been great about working on my Daily Checklist lately. I attack it each morning with a passion. I have been consciously trying to take advantage of each minute of the day. Today, while sitting in the dentist's chair (dreading the drill), I thought, ''Hey! Why sit here and waste time? Surely there's something I can do in my head.'' And *voilà*! I thought of ''thinking thin.'' My eyes were shut anyway, so I started concentrating on thinness.

I visualized it all: the happy, thin experiences of traveling, being Rose Festival princess, turning guys' heads, swimming, dancing—it was wonderful. Then I thought, ''Rosemary, you'll probably be here for another hour. Why not go for broke?'' So right there, in the dentist's chair, I became 125 pounds, put on the daringest, skimpiest, most provocative little teddy you ever did see and proceeded to seduce my husband. At one point, I almost choked on my own laughter. Whatever would Dr. Cantwell think if he knew my thoughts at that moment? After fifteen years of fat, I must admit, it's more than a little exciting to contemplate . . . dare I say it? . . . sex as a skinny me. An uninhibited me. I'm going to need a new closet built—for my sleepwear alone!

The crazy kicker here is this: I was so fat, I barely fit into the dentist's chair. My hips were hanging over the armrests in a most disgusting way. I cringed when I sat down, and, like Silly Putty, had to kind of melt into that ridiculously small seat. I swear, the people who make those chairs must think that if you're more than twenty pounds overweight, you're immune to cavities!

What a miserable addiction food is. I'm sure there are times when alcoholics or drug addicts are so far into never-never land that they are unaware of their misery. They have to come down off their self-induced high before they realize how miserable they are. Eating chocolate does not wipe away my pain, it does not send me to never-never land. Of course, I have no desire to exchange addictions with a heroin user, but it would be nice if there were a harmless way to forget my fat and hide my degradation for a while—even if it were only from myself.

Thursday was awful. I need to write about it, so I will never forget. I've been in a deep state of depression; morbid obesity, a messy house, severe debt, and seven baby-sitting kids a day add up to severe depression every time. But, hey, I have the power to eliminate two of the four. My body is my own. (Though I'm not exactly thrilled to claim it at this particular time!) And it *is* physically possible to clean my house. In fact, if I would lose weight, it would be easier to clean the house, because I'd have more energy. And if I were skinny, I could become a famous movie star and make lots of money and . . . yes! *All* my problems would be solved. Okay, so the movie star idea is a little ludicrous (I'll let that one go), but at least half my problems would be solved.

Being off my diet is hideous. Mentally and physically. I get sick to my stomach from eating pure garbage all day long, and I also feel sluggish and blah and exhausted. (Probably a result of the horrendous sugar overdose.) The physical reaction to terrible eating habits is extremely negative, but the mental and emotional consequences are even more devastating. My mind and soul seem to ingest the garbage, too. My sense of humor shrivels up and dies. Nothing is funny, cute, or clever. All hope vanishes. My love for family, for life itself, diminishes. My very soul, the essence of me, shrinks to a state of near nothingness. I experience an emptiness inside so acute that I feel like a mere shell—a big, fat, ugly, unloved, and unwanted shell.

Thursday, I felt a horrible weight on my chest, like a wave crashing over me. I kept finding myself gulping for air. I kept having to grab on to something, just to maintain balance.

Did you ever see that delightful Walt Disney movie *Pollyanna*? In one scene, the preacher is perched behind the pulpit with an extremely stern look on his face. He almost scowls at the congregation and then suddenly blasts out at them in a growly voice: "Death comes unexpectedly!" His intensity nearly knocks you out of your chair! Well, that's how my depression waves come—unexpectedly. As when I was happily doing my laundry, pleased to be on my last load, and *whammo!* Suddenly, I was submerged in despair. I could be doing anything; those waves came all day long.

However (and this is important), I was desperate for the depression to go away. I didn't want to sink so far down that I would drown for who knows how many days. I wanted out and I fought back. After each horrid wave of despair, I would mentally cry out, "Oh, please, God, help it to go away. I want to feel happy. I want to accomplish something today. Only I can pull myself out of this, but you can give me extra strength. Please help me now!"

I survived Thursday. Thank goodness Allen took all the children to Matthew's Cub Scout pack meeting that night. For one hour I had no one but me to take care of. It had been months since I'd had an entire hour to myself.

Wednesday, June 3, 1987
244 pounds

I talk of my diet constantly. I think of future events, not in terms of dates, but in terms of pounds. Not "We go to the beach on June twenty-sixth," but "Only twenty more pounds, and we go to the beach."

It amazes me that I willingly give the needle on the scale such incredible power over me. We fatties all know that it doesn't really matter how much we weigh, only how we look and feel. If I could find a scale to weigh me in at 110 pounds, I'd still be overweight. I'd still have fat rolls around my middle. I'd still hate the way I look. Yet somehow, that nasty little needle does have an impact on how I feel about myself.

I found out today that fat people aren't the only ones suffering from "fear of needles." My friend Cindy has no visible fat on her body. Yesterday, I stopped by her house for a visit. She immediately informed me that she was thrilled because she had just lost ten pounds without even dieting. "Now I can tuck in my blouse! I feel great. See, aren't I looking better?" She twirled around in front of me.

It was a cruel twist of fate that brought her husband out of the bathroom at that precise moment. Oh, cruel, cruel twist. "Cindy, I put a new battery in the scale. The other one was getting weak." Yes, Cindy quit twirling. Cindy quit smiling. Cindy's eyes opened wide in disbelief. See Cindy run to the bathroom. See Cindy step on the scale. Hear Cindy's quick intake of breath. See Cindy come slowly out of the bathroom. See Cindy's blouse untucked. Poor, poor Cindy. And yet . . .

Cindy was the same weight she had been only seconds before. But now, feeling fat, she could no longer tuck in her blouse. All this because of some dumb needle on some dumb scale. Crazy, isn't it?

Then there's Rosanne. She and I go back a long way. She struggles with her weight, too. Once, while conversing about our fat, we both cracked up over the story of her "skinny dress." I'm not kidding; that's what she called it—her skinny dress. From the first moment she tried it on, she felt sleek and sexy. Rosanne said, "When I looked in the mirror, I thought I looked practically thin. I kinda vamped my way out into the living room, where my husband was reading the paper. I took what I considered to be an alluring pose and then stood there waiting for him to notice how good I looked. He didn't even glance up from his paper. I cleared my throat a few times, and he finally asked if I wanted something. Trying to sound a little coy, I asked, 'Is it just me, or do I look almost skinny in this dress?'

"He lifted his eyes from his paper and gave me one quick appraisal. 'It's just you.' Boy, was I shot down. But I felt so skinny in that dress that I was sure he was somehow wrong.

"I asked my daughter, who was within earshot in the kitchen, 'Honey, what do you think?'

"It took her only a second to check me out. 'Sorry, Mom,

Dad's right. It *is* just you.' The crazy thing is, I still like to wear that dress. Despite their responses, it makes me feel skinny.''

Rosanne and I were practically rolling on the floor in hysterics by the time she finished telling that story. It was so stupid. A *skinny dress*. Can you believe that . . . course, I *did* have a pair of ''magic shoes'' once. No, I'm not kidding. They were magic. They were the cutest, voguest little things, made from a white, lacy material. And I swear to you, when I put them on, I *became skinnier*.

Now, I have large feet. I have never owned a pair of shoes that didn't look something like oars for a rowboat . . . except for those magic shoes. They were darling just to look at. It always amazed me that my feet could even slip into them. In fact, that's how I first knew they were magic. I returned to the shoe store to buy all the rest that they had in stock, but there were none left. Dang it!

Wednesday, June 10, 1987
239 pounds

I weigh 239 pounds today. When I lose an additional:

2 pounds (237),   Jay will go to an AA meeting. (He promised to, if I lost 25 pounds.)

7 pounds (232),   Mom will give me $30 for a 30-pound loss.

9 pounds (230),   I will try on all my clothes to see what fits me.

15 pounds (224),   I will need to lose only 99 more pounds.

19 pounds (220),   I will ride my bike.

27 pounds (212),	Mom will give me $20 (for a total 50-pound loss).
29 pounds (210),	I will weigh what I did when I became pregnant with Tyler. I will try on all my clothes again.
40 pounds (199),	I'll be in the 100s.
44 pounds (195),	I will weigh less than I have in over ten years.
46 pounds (193),	I'll be halfway through dieting; I'll have lost 69 pounds.
49 pounds (190),	I will wear hats.
69 pounds (170),	I will try on all my clothes.
79 pounds (160),	I will be three-fourths through dieting; I'll have lost 102 pounds.
84 pounds (155),	I will weigh less than Allen!
89 pounds (150),	I will be lower than I've been in sixteen years. I will try on all my clothes.
96 pounds (143),	I will weigh what I did the day I was married.
109 pounds (130),	I will weigh less than I have in nineteen years—less than I ever have as an adult.

Thursday, June 18, 1987
239 pounds

Let's be honest. Extremely obese people either have a humongous rear end, thunder thighs, or a never-ending stomach. Some, sorry to say, have all three! After the poor body has enlarged itself as much as possible in a vaguely human way, there is no place to expand but downward. Gravity takes its toll. The body erupts further, in an elephantlike way—with the fat hanging in layers. Just hanging there! Horrible, disgusting fat!

Well, folks, when fat people try to run or exercise with all this elephant flab, look out! They discover what self-torture is all about. I nearly beat myself to death—with the fat from my own body—when I first started to exercise. And it was almost impossible to do a simple curl-up because there was such a disgusting amount of lard around my middle.

Jumping jacks are difficult to describe. The noise alone is repulsive. Jump-*slap*-jump-*slap*. My fat stomach actually spanks the top of my legs. Ouch! How did I ever do this to my body, to my life? Can you imagine how good it felt one day to realize the "slapping" sound was less intense? (This subject is so disgusting that I can hardly believe I'm going to print this entry about myself.)

Tuesday, July 7, 1987
243 pounds

I haven't cracked my workbook for twenty days. And guess what? A four-pound gain. Woe is me. I've been on vacation, and it's always hard to maintain control while traveling. Why should a vacation from work mean a vacation from my diet? Somewhere in my distant past, I came to associate vacation time with one continual orgy of food.

As a child, I never had any dream vacations. When I heard my friends say they were going to Disneyland, I would marvel. Going to Disneyland and going to the moon were synonymous to me. I distinctly remember thinking, "Wow, I didn't know that kid was a millionaire!" But we did go camping a lot and had exceptional fun. As I reflect back on my camping experiences, I can see the seeds of the if-this-is-a-vacation-we-must-eat-like-pigs syndrome. And we did.

Our first stop on any trip always occurred shortly after leaving our driveway. Our old, homemade camper-truck would pull into the parking lot of some neighborhood store, and five or six of us children would pile out and head straight for the candy counter. We'd each pick our favorite "poison" and pack back into the truck. It wasn't until we had a candy bar in our hands that we felt officially on our way. If we were going any significant distance, there would be several such stops. Sometimes at an ice cream store, sometimes at a bakery. Not one of us ever refused one sweet thing. Not one of us was ever too full or not hungry. *Not* and *hungry* were two words that never were spoken together in my family.

Mom always packed an abundance of sweets and goodies for any trip. I mean, who in the world could have fun without them? She baked cookies by the dozens. (Of course, she practically had to stand guard over them with a gun before we left home!) She baked her famous applesauce cake for every trip.

On one camping trip, Dad sneaked up in the middle of the night for a sweet fix. (When the need for sweets arose . . . so did he.) Mom was sound asleep when Dad started rooting around in the food boxes, trying to find something that would hit the spot. He knew Mom would be upset with him for doing so, but he cut into the applesauce cake. Now, no red-blooded, still-breathing child in my family could bear to see anyone eat alone, especially if that someone was eating a piece of Mom's applesauce cake. We sneaked out of bed and asked Dad for a piece. If too much cake was missing, he knew he'd be in big trouble, so he told us to go ask Mom. We peeked our heads into the tent and whispered, "Can we have some applesauce cake?"

Now, Mother was a mighty snorer. People hate to hear

that about themselves, but she could outsnore anyone, except maybe Dad. When we oh-so-quietly whispered our plea for cake, she was in the middle of an intense snoring episode. With a good imagination, it was conceivable to hear, "*Hoooonk* . . . sure. *Hoooonk* . . . sure." We skipped merrily back to Dad, looked him straight in the eyes, and innocently said, "Mom said, 'Sure'!" And we "*hoooonk* . . . sure-d" our way through the whole cake.

It was probably the only time any of us children ever got the best of Dad. Oh boy, was Mom fuming when she woke up. Not only was the cake eaten without her permission, she hadn't tasted one little bite of it! Mom loved her sweets, too.

When we explained the circumstances surrounding our request to Mom for cake, she didn't see the humor in it. Fortunately, time has softened the memory and "*hoooonk* . . . sure" is one of our favorite family jokes.

Time, however, has not softened the memory of how Dad would sneak . . . take . . . steal . . . our cans of pop while we were camping. Yes, he was a real stinker about it. Mom would buy a whole case of pop. Each of us would get "x" number of cans. Dad would inevitably drink all of his the first day and then sneak . . . take . . . steal . . . from his own children. In order to assure that your pop was drunk by you, and you alone, you had to drink yours faster than Dad drank his. It was a dirty trick, especially to me.

You see, I have always been an avid reader. One of my favorite vacation activities was to lie in the shade on a hot summer day and read a book. Put a cold can of pop in my hand, and I was in heaven. So I liked to stretch my pops out to the last day of our camping trip. Hard to do with Dad around. Sometimes I would hide them and put one in the cooler shortly before I wanted to drink it, but even then it wasn't safe. I lost many a pop within minutes after trying to chill it. It was especially irritating to lose one of my precious cans to some neighboring camper Dad was trying to impress with his generosity. Gee whiz, if he wanted to be "big man on campus," he could have given away his own treats. The stinker!

Yes, I learned young that on vacations you start out with sweets, you bring tons of sweets, you eat your share, and you eat it fast. After writing this, I'm going to make a conscious effort to never encourage the same behavior in my children. At least I never have to worry about Allen sneaking their treats. The dear man wouldn't dream of pulling my Dad's bum trick. I often tell the children when Allen isn't around, "Okay, you guys, this is the last piece of chicken, the last cookie, the last peach, etc. I'm saving it for Daddy. He'll ask if you want some, so pretend you don't. I want him to have it."

After recalling those thoughts, I realize it's no wonder I ate like a pig on our recent vacation. I had planned to be good. I brought my scale and workbook with me. I *intended* to do my diet faithfully. But stupid me! Now I have to lose that same stupid four pounds one more time!

I can't gain any more weight back. I'm too miserable. And I spend too much money on junk food. I deliberately stop at different little neighborhood stores so that no single cashier will know how much I eat. Isn't that ridiculous? Every sane, breathing person knows I eat like a Sumo wrestler! Except maybe doctors, and it seems doctors will believe almost any lie a fat person can concoct to hide her eating habits.

I was recently talking with a doctor at Kaiser. Allen was with me. I do not recall why weight was brought up, but when I admitted to the doctor I was fat because I eat like a pig, he registered absolute shock. I told him, "Do you know how many heavy-duty calories it takes to maintain this shape? If someone as fat as I am tells you she is eating only green salads and chicken legs twice a day, believe me, Doctor, she is lying!" His eyes squinted that sort of ahhhh-I-see-the-light look as he nodded his head up and down in a knowing way. He almost spoke to himself when he said, "I wondered about that." Allen and I both exploded with laughter. I tell you, in some areas a doctor's degree is no substitute for experience.

Sometimes, the thought of dedicating myself to a diet, of saying good-bye to "old friends," puts me into a panic. It makes me feel trapped and anxious and paranoid and you-can't-make-me-I-can-eat-anything-I-want-ish. Today I'm too weak to commit to a diet, but I can commit to doing my Daily Checklist. Go, Rosemary, go! Hip, hip . . . away!

Friday, July 10, 1987
239 pounds

I can't believe my willpower is so thin sometimes. Ha! Would that my body were so thin and my willpower a little more chubby! Case in point. For several days, I had been perfect on my diet; then I attended my friend Kathy Mueller's bridal shower.

If only the hostess had served just cake and punch. I was prepared for cake and punch. I was ready to say casually, "No, thanks." But no, she had to go and serve a complete gourmet meal. I was not prepared for a complete gourmet meal! I fought myself for a full three seconds. Then I sauntered over to the buffet table, restraining myself from breaking into a dead run, holding in my stomach, trying to look thin, yet dying to indulge.

"I will have only a couple of deviled eggs," I told myself in a vague, noncommittal sort of way. Ha! I should have stopped and mentally hyped myself up: "Eggs, Rosemary, allow yourself two egg halves. That will be a special treat. Two egg halves, two egg halves, two egg halves." But no! I stupidly marched headlong into temptation. As I ogled tray after tray of delicious food, my hand reached out, unbidden, for a small scoop of this, a tiny helping of that.

I couldn't believe it. By the time I came out of my hypnotic trance, my plate was *full*. Two egg halves, my eye! I ate at least eight (if you consider the ones I popped into my mouth, whole, at the serving table). "Get a grip, girl! Where is your pride?" I was so ashamed of myself, a big fat woman eating whole egg halves while heaping her plate with tons more. But I proceeded to make up for the last few days of dieting. I had two bran muffins, three slices of banana bread, chicken salad, a large serving of guacamole and bean dip with chips, six olives, and fruit salad—thank goodness the hostess didn't serve dessert! Actually, I would have been better off if she had, for when I left the shower, I felt like a caged tiger. I felt almost crazy. As I walked to the car, I suddenly knew why. I wasn't through eating!

I wanted, I needed, I craved something sweet! Bingo! I almost felt relief. Hey, I'd gone this far; why not stop and get a candy bar? *A* candy bar? As in "one"? Suuuure! I ate the Twix bar and three-fifths of a new chocolate bar on the way home. The new one was less than terrific. I would never buy it again. It had five segments. But did I stop at one? No. Even though I wasn't too fond of it, I managed to struggle through two more segments before I said audibly, "I don't even *like* this candy." I put the last two segments back in the sack, back with my extra-large Baby Ruth and extra-large Butterfinger. (They sure named them right: you buy extra-large, you *become* extra-large!)

Well, I downed those two extra-large bars immediately upon entering the house and locking myself in my bedroom. I did my usual hide-the-evidence trick. I put all the candy wrappers back in the sack and twisted it so it looked like garbage; no one would ever look inside. I was about to toss the evidence, when suddenly I thought of those two segments of candy that I hadn't eaten, that I didn't even like. I had chosen to chuck them when I still had an extra-large Baby Ruth and an extra-large Butterfinger in my hungry little hands. But now that I was candyless, it was another story.

"Maybe it wasn't such a bad candy bar after all. And I really shouldn't waste it. I should at least offer it to one of my children." *Suuuure* I'd give it to one of my children. I reopened the sack, retrieved the slightly squished candy, and carefully rewadded the sack to cover my tracks. (Thieves are less careful than I!)

I didn't eat the last two segments of candy that night. I walked into the kitchen, where my children were waiting for me to play a game of Clue. I put the chocolate on top of the fridge. I'd finished my food binge for the night. So why didn't I throw away that stupid, not-so-tasty piece of hell and misery? I don't know.

I visited Debbie the next day and had a green salad with low-calorie dressing. I told Mom and Debbie to be good on their diets. Yet, even as I walked out the door of Debbie's house, I knew my fate. The second I'd said "diet," a picture of those two slightly squished pieces of chocolate candy flashed before my eyes. Before I had started the car, my mind was made up. I drove home, strode straight to the kitchen, and made a beeline for the fridge. I popped those two sections of candy into my mouth faster than a junkie pops pills. And then—and this just kills me—I made up some pastry as fast as I could.

So, do you think I am sick? Unbalanced? Out of control? Or (D), all of the above? When I phoned Melissa later that day, we talked a little fat. We always do. She told me how hard it is not to eat sweets when she makes them herself. Then she admitted she was nervous about making some chocolate chip cookies for a party at work the next day. I, myself, felt like a runaway train. I knew that if I didn't pull the emergency brake soon, I was going to crash hard. So I summoned up the courage to blurt out, "Okay, Melissa, if you eat *one* of those chocolate chip cookies, you have to pay me five dollars. And if I eat *one* more bite of food today, I'll pay you five dollars." Crazily enough, it worked. I had desperately needed something to stop me. I didn't have the five dollars and I knew I couldn't lie to Melissa, so instead of eating, I just kept repeating, "Today is the *fattest* day of the rest of my life."

Saturday, July 11, 1987
239 pounds

It's been unusually hard to keep my mind off food today. I have to record my own motivational tapes, both "night tapes" and "day tapes." I need to hear hype regularly. I need it desperately. I need to listen to it during the day as I'm putting on my makeup or vacuuming or washing dishes. What a wonderful way to get motivated while I'm doing my daily chores. And I need a tape I can listen to each night to help me keep on the straight and narrow diet trail the following day.

Thursday, July 23, 1987
239 pounds

I am consumed with the thought of losing these extra 100 pounds. It's these darned last 100 pounds that have made me so miserable. (Yes, that's a joke! You know how you always hear those disgustingly skinny ladies saying in their high-pitched voices: "Oh my, these last three pounds are such a nuisance!" I want to push them into a swimming pool when they're dressed in their fanciest clothes!)

Today, Debbie and I thought of a new idea. We call it the "Buck a Bite" program. Today, just this one day, Debbie and I agreed to eat absolutely, positively, *exactly* what we listed on our Daily Menu. We decided to pay a "Buck a Bite" for eating anything not listed on it! I could lose my house over that one!

Okay. This is it. I write it here in black and white. I am *positive* I am going to do it. I am going to lose weight. I am finally going to dissolve this blubber. Melt this butter. Sizzle this Crisco. Hang on, Allen, I'll be voluptuous yet!

Monday, July 27, 1987
236 pounds

Monday morning. A fresh, new start. I love new starts. New chances. And this morning I'm in critical need of one. Last night I was screaming out of control at my husband and son. My behavior was inexcusable and I am bitterly ashamed. But the soothing balm of this fresh morning air reminds me that like the new day, I can start over.

Today I weigh less than I have since Tyler was born. Tomorrow I break the "pound barrier." When I begin to get close to my previous lowest weight, I swear my body goes into red alert and starts fighting any additional weight loss. My mind is my main enemy at this point. Part of it starts this rationale: "You are looking so much better these days. Why, you're looking as good as you have in years. Go ahead, have a treat. You deserve it." It sounds absurd, but often getting down to "the lowest weight I've been in years" (even though that amount is eighty-some pounds more than my ideal weight) signals the end of my diet. So I am more than a little anxious to break the . . . *pound barrier*!

Wednesday, August 5, 1987
235 pounds

Tomorrow we're having company for dinner. *Company for dinner*. Three words that fill me with happy anticipation— and, at the same time, fill me with foreboding. You see, I am a marvelous cook. I think I have magic fingers. Everything I touch turns out incredibly delicious. It is almost impossible for me to whip up a batch of anything without eating half the dough and another half of the finished product. Therefore, when company comes, and I make some of my yummiest recipes, I delight in the eating but burn in hell over the resulting extra calories. However, when I plan ahead and commit myself to no nibbles, telling Allen to monitor me, I do pretty well.

Today I make my stand against the temptations and horrors of tomorrow. I will not eat one piece of my divine homemade bread or one spoonful of potato salad. I will not eat a bite of cake or lick one dab of frosting off my fingers. I will have a green salad with low-calorie dressing, Sugar Free Jell-O, and that is all.

Monday, August 10, 1987
235 pounds

Jon Tyler's birthday! In nine short months I gained ninety pounds. Today, one year later, I've lost sixty-five of those pounds. It doesn't take a mathematician to figure I'm up twenty-five pounds from when I became pregnant. Now, twenty-five pounds is livable, especially for someone as tall as I am. The problem is that I began my pregnancy eighty-five pounds overweight! Will it ever end? I must get out of this whirlpool. It keeps me going around in circles. I lose a few pounds here and there, then get sucked down into the fear, depression, and self-hatred of being fat, which always results in an amazing, five-pound-or-more instant gain. Then I throw out a line and climb—

Thursday, September 3, 1987
236 pounds

Climb where? Well, I'll tell you where I'm climbing today: *I'm climbing out! Out*, you hear me? I am so tired of being disgusted with me. Hating me. Disappointed with me. Rosemary is somewhere deep inside this "incredible hulk." She still lives and breathes, loves and cares, laughs and cries. She is yet capable of accomplishing something worthwhile with her life. I've been like a huge blob of flesh lately— without much purpose. I'm not happy. I look and feel like a giant slug!

Two weeks ago, I met Alice again. She was one of the Rose Festival princesses on the court with me in 1970. Like the last time, I felt miserably uncomfortable meeting her. She was as thin as ever, looking incredibly chic. I looked and felt exactly like what I was: an old, fat housewife. My stomach hung out like a hippo. I was wearing thongs. My hair was pulled back in a barrette (as if I were cute and thin enough to wear ponytails), and it was slightly in need of washing. I didn't have on as much makeup as I usually do.

I rarely step outside my front door unless I look the best I can, because at my weight, even my best is frightful! But wouldn't you know it, whenever I'm at my worst, I manage to meet the classiest people from my past! I felt a new wave of humiliation crush down on me each second that I stood there and talked to her. But she was sweet. When she asked me to come to the next Rose Festival reunion, I felt she meant it. I felt she genuinely wanted me to know it didn't matter if I *am* fat. Thank you, Alice. You made me feel better.

After a few minutes of conversation, she began telling me her problems—critical problems. What? A thin, glamorous person with something to beef about? (Why, always, do I find food adjectives coming to my mind?) She had been separated for two years and was finally deciding if she would officially file for a divorce. Two years. Her husband had an affair. Now, that's irony for you. There I was, standing in torturous misery, wishing I could sink into a hole in the ground, despising myself for looking like a fat, unclassy slob. I was coveting her thin body, her stylish clothes, her up-to-the-minute hair-do. Then, suddenly, my heart ached for her. Alice's husband had become involved with another woman. For all my meanness and grotesque obesity, Allen is 100 percent faithful to me.

I doubt that Alice would want to trade problems with me, but I certainly would never trade with her. Give up my wonderful, loyal husband? Give up my five beautiful, precious children? For a skinny body? No, thanks. Besides, this is the fattest day of the rest of my life—so I *can* have it all. I can have a loyal husband, five children, *and* a thin body. Though I won't be "skinny" tomorrow, I will be skinnier. This is the last time I start. This is it. To the end. Not the bitter end, but the *better* end.

Thursday, September 24, 1987
244 pounds

So many things to write about. Failures. Problems. Frustrations. Depression. So little hope or happiness. Until yesterday. Yesterday, I felt a tiny glimmer. I felt an old feeling of excitement stir slightly within me, yawn, stretch a little, and open one eye. That exhilarating feeling of—is there a word for maybe-this-misery-will-not-go-on-forever-after-all? I guess there is only one word for it: hope.

Without hope, life is merely a matter of marking time. And somehow, somewhere, I lost precious hope. I've lost lots of stuff in my life, but I've never lost anything half as well as I've lost hope. It's a horrible, empty feeling.

Each day is merely a series of hours. Cooking, cleaning, changing diapers, chauffeuring children, answering phones. No joy, no fun. Only a kind of dull awareness that I'm alive. A horrible feeling in the morning that I must suffer through another whole day before I can drown myself in sleep again. Oh, wonderful sleep. At least there I can escape for a few hours from the total misery of reality, of life. It's a pleasant break from the monotony of existing, the real highlight of my day.

But enough talk of depression! I'd rather think of that feeling I experienced yesterday, of excitement stirring within. If I look hard, if I strain and squint, I can see a tiny pinpoint of light at the end of my tunnel. That's hope. Hope trying to shine through. I'm too apprehensive to get excited, but I'm smiling as I write these words, and that's a good sign!

I have to get this saggy, baggy fat off my beautiful body. I have to find me again. "Oh, where, oh, where has my little bod gone? Oh, where, oh, where can she be? With her thin, pretty neck and her long, sexy legs—oh, where, oh, where can she be?" I miss her so much.

Tuesday, November 3, 1987
248 pounds

I had to write today because I can't go on another second like this. My misery is so all-consuming, I can hardly breathe. I'm too humiliated to leave my house, and thoughts of suicide dance like demons through my mind. Besides my emotional duress, I am having chest pains and dizzy spells. My knees creak like an old rocking chair every time I climb stairs. My stomach is constantly churning. I want to feel healthy and energetic again!

I'm accomplishing *nothing* these days. I'm always exhausted from lugging around over 100 pounds of "butter" everywhere I go. Over 100 pounds of butter! I cannot put that wretched butter down, even if I have to climb stairs, run to comfort an injured child, or waddle to the kitchen to look for something yummy!

I've been "looking for something yummy" for as long as I can remember. Once, years ago, when Mom and Dad were out, my siblings and I were sitting around watching TV. Suddenly, we were all overcome by the urge for something sweet to eat. Let's face it, we had been conditioned to be chomping on *something* whenever we were in front of the TV.

We scoured those cupboards as if searching for a last meal. As always, there was not one cookie or candy or pastry to be had. We were desperate. What could we do? Someone spied a box of Jell-O and came up with the unique idea of dividing it into equal shares. We then used toothpicks to lick and dip into the Jell-O powder. It made a rather tasty treat.

I remember that incident with two distinctly sad feelings. First, we had quite a debate as to whether we should or should not open that box of Jell-O. We were concerned that Mom might get mad at us for using it up. We finally took the chance that it would be okay if we were willing to pay for a new box later on. We all had to commit a grand total of three cents apiece. Gee whiz, three cents! It makes me sad to remember being worried over an eighteen-cent box of Jell-O.

It also makes me sad that the need to eat overtook our young lives. I vividly remember the emotions of that night. We *had* to find something to eat, or the whole evening would be ruined. Why did food have to play such an important role in our happiness? Why does food continue to do so today? I hate it. This very moment, I am toying with the idea of making a trip to the store solely to buy some mouthwatering, chocolate-covered malt balls.

I discovered this fabulous treat a few days ago. In the bulk foods section. Oh, heaven! Oh, hell! We are not talking plain old Whoppers here. These things are in a whole different category. The chocolate is thick and rich and melts in your mouth like some life-giving ambrosia. I actually daydream about those glorious, chocolate-coated little balls of misery. I visualize popping one into my mouth and then sinking into the wondrous sensation of creamy, thick, sweet chocolate, followed by the satisfying crunch of the now uncovered malt ball.

Someday, maybe I will reach deep into my past and discover I don't like chocolate after all. Nah, no such luck.

Monday, January 25, 1988
261 pounds

Over two and a half months. No entry! I weigh more than I ever have, except when I was pregnant. After Tyler was born (August 1986), I settled in at 280 pounds. Insane. Oh, misery. Then shortly afterward, my sister Debbie and I decided to be buddies and help each other burn off the lard! After many false starts and lots of true stops, I finally reached a low of 232. Felt—if not human—at least able to bend over.

Then I lost all control, and I'm up to 261 this morning. I reached 265 a few days ago. It was a nightmare! With my eyes bulging out of my head in horror, I calmed down with respect to food for a few days. I didn't diet, but I calmed down a little. I gritted my teeth and bravely drove past all the drive-through food places, the convenience stores, and pastry shops. Yes, that's calming down. Of course, I *made* myself some brownies and the filling to a super-rich chocolate mousse pie. I felt absurdly generous when I gave my son a small piece of a brownie. Gee whiz! One small piece of brownie. That means I ate all the rest myself. I ate some three dozen brownies all by myself. I hate me.

I can hardly bring myself to spell out what I am about to say. But almost as a punishment, I'm going to make myself write about mother pigs.

Have you ever been to the state fair? Remember those huge, disgusting blobs with the cute little piglets nestling around? It was hideous, but I kept visualizing that scene the last time I made love. No, I didn't envision the cute little piglets. I saw, instead, the gross-big-fat mother pigs.

Allen and I were out of town in a beautiful, romantic hotel room. We had just eaten dinner, and I felt especially full. There I was, 265 pounds of distended, misshapen flesh, a veritable mother pig. I hope I will never forget how totally disgusted I was with myself that night. Poor Allen. *I* never would have stayed married to me!

Lately, I can't sit down without feeling my stomach in my lap, six inches of flab squished out over the top of my legs whenever I'm seated. When I hold Tyler at church, and he drops a toy, it's very difficult to bend over to pick it up. My stomach stops me. The sheer lard around my middle keeps me from reaching the floor. It's distressing to bend over in my chair and not be able to pick up an object right at my feet. I end up having to kind of bob up and down a few times. Then, finally, like a spring, I can stretch far enough and grab the object off the floor. (Oh, curse you, all you skinny, small-waisted ladies who effortlessly bend over to retrieve your tots' toys! Sometimes I hate every last one of you!)

Yesterday, I listened to a conversation on the radio about a heavyweight boxing champion who stands six feet tall and weighs 220 pounds! Yup, the radio announcer said it with an exclamation point—a whopping 220 pounds! And I sat in my car wishing *I* weighed only 220 pounds. Here's the real clincher: I was sitting in my car, waiting outside our little neighborhood grocery store for my son to come out with the three candy bars I had sent him after. Waiting for my three candy bars, wishing I weighed only 220 pounds. Let me make the pathos of the scene even more graphic by pointing out that I sent my son in for the candy bars because I was too chagrined to get out of my car. Too fat to want to hoist my bulk out and back again.

I am determined that I will *never* again have to wish I weighed less than a heavyweight boxing champion. I am determined that I will *never* again have to hate sitting with my stomach in my lap. I am determined that I will *never* again have to feel like a mother pig. Never.

Sunday, March 6, 1988
272 pounds

Two hundred seventy-two pounds, the most I've ever weighed without being pregnant. Two hundred seventy-two pounds! Those words are overwhelming. The bulges and ripples on my body are unbelievable. They are distressingly akin to those of a full-grown hippo!

The energy it takes to merely walk around my house is more than I can handle. I am in a constant state of exhaustion! The wrenching noise my knees make as I climb stairs is terrifying. The time has come. I must take action. I'm afraid I'm going to die if I don't. Sometimes my heart hurts, and I keep having dizzy spells. I'm scared of dying, while I'm thinking of ways to kill myself because I'm so miserable! I have lived so many years so distressed with myself that my depression alone is life-threatening. And it's my own, fat fault. My own, out-of-control eating. My own, what-can-I-stuff-into-my-mouth-next behavior.

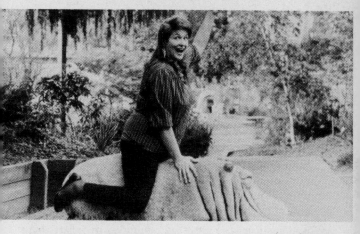

August 1990, 200 pounds. It was great to take this crazy pose *on* a hippo instead of feeling *like* one.

I wish I could fully describe the ugliness of obesity. I'm sitting here—oh, sitting is the worst! I have this huge, blubbery mass of flesh extending out from under my bosom and falling, hanging, onto my lap. My lungs feel all squished up. I never get a good, deep breath. Fat-filled rolls of flesh slap my body if I move fast. I feel the fat on my arms shake as I barely move around. My arms are so puffed up that they don't hang straight down at my sides; they flare out—like a full skirt. I feel the fat on my chin jiggle as I talk or turn my head.

I feel something like a split personality. I am the perfect example of two people trying frantically to live together in one body. Only my problem is that my body ballooned up—stretched itself—to accommodate the other person. True schizophrenics share only the mind. I don't like the other person with whom I am sharing my body. I hate her. She is mean and angry. She is impatient. She is frustrated. She is everything I don't like about me. I am determined to get rid of her in the cruel way she deserves: I'm going to starve her to death! (I like that thought!)

I have filled in my Weight-Loss Goal Calendar and taken my measurements. I can't let it depress me, but it is major-disgusting. You know the famous, hourglass, 36–24–36 figure? Well, how does this grab you? 51½–53–59! For crying out loud—I'm a triangle! This *is* the fattest day of the rest of my life!

Monday, March 7, 1988
269 pounds

It is impossible to look at myself in the mirror without feeling tremendous disgust. I am totally mortified by what I have allowed myself to become. But when my fat directly results in emotional and physical pain to one of my children, my misery becomes unbearable.

Jennifer is in the seventh grade. Her teachers all love her. I am constantly getting good reports from them. She has earned straight A's, and I am very proud of that. But even more important to me is the fact that she has received all E's for "excellence" in behavioral skills: Is Courteous, Shows Self-Control, Respects Property of Others, Co-operates With Others, etc. Yet with that kind of report card, she has still experienced the year from hell.

In the last few months, a group of students Jennifer calls "The Nasty Nine" has evolved into a menacing gang. They have singled out Jennifer as their target. For five months, poor little Jenny has endured their cruel remarks, their foul names, their nasty gestures, and their daily threats to her health. For five months she has been pushed, hit, kicked, and tripped. For five months she has had her hair yanked and her possessions snatched. This kind of torment, *every day for five months*!

I only recently found out how serious it was. I knew Jenny

had been unhappy at school, but it was one of those things I put on the back burner to worry about later. Since she knew I would try to stop it, she had been afraid to tell me too much about the problem. She was terrified that The Nasty Nine would become even more violent toward her.

Jennifer was right about my trying to stop it. I talked to Jennifer's three teachers and the school principal. They all agreed that Jennifer was a victim of jealousy. I also called four other girls at Jenny's school. They affirmed everything Jennifer had said about the gang and added even more injustices that they had observed.

Rather than taking the advice of the police to press charges that would lead to the arrest of the gang members, I wrote a letter to Jennifer's schoolteachers, her principal, and to the parents of the nine girls. The principal was finally forced into acknowledging the problem because I now had complaints, in writing, from five different people against The Nasty Nine.

I let the school administrators know, in no uncertain terms, that they had a problem to work out. They needed to figure out how to handle juvenile delinquents. (No one even told these girls they committed illegal, expellable offenses. The girls never even wrote Jennifer a note of apology.) My daughter deserves to be able to go to school without fear of daily physical violence.

What does all this have to do with hating myself for my weight? It is hard to explain adequately. Several months before I was aware of Jennifer's intense misery at school, I had experienced similar crudities and rudeness from these very girls. As I was walking down the hall at school, driving home from school, or waiting in my car to pick up my children from school, these very girls yelled out swear words at me. They gave me the finger. They made ugly faces at me. Merely because I was Jennifer's mother. That should have made me realize that something horrible was happening to Jennifer.

I am now conscience-stricken because I did not respond to the very first young brat who violated the school language code. I can't help blaming myself for this thing escalating to such hideous magnitude for Jennifer. But when you weigh over 270 pounds, your self-esteem is shot. It is difficult to confront young, skinny, sexy teenagers when you feel like an old blimp; I knew I was just a big, fat joke to them. And it is burdensome to lug my near 300-pound physique out of my car to nab those juvenile delinquents and drag them into the principal's office. Even in one of my angriest, bravest moods, it is nearly impossible to march into a principal's office to declare that certain girls called me a fat ————. After all, I *am* fat! Had I been thin, I would have had those girls in deep trouble long ago, but I was intimidated by them. Oh! It makes me livid just thinking about it. I refuse to be in such a horrible position again. I want my freedom back.

I am sorry that my obesity, my own out-of-control eating, kept me from protecting you from suffering those many atrocities. I am so sorry, my darling Jenny.

Wednesday, March 9, 1988
264 pounds

I will never weigh 272 pounds again! I'm ahead of my Weight-Loss Goal Calendar. It feels divine! I love life when I'm dieting. It's not only because I'm eating less and losing weight, it's that I've taken control of *me* again. I haven't been yelling as much. I'm no longer experiencing acute paranoia. I'm not as frustrated, angry, or depressed. I see my successes more, little though they might be. I feel hope for the future.

Yesterday I went shopping. I bravely (or could it be stupidly?) bought some candy for Jenny to give to her "secret pal" in her church class, and I didn't buy any for myself. I wasn't tempted because I kept telling myself, "I want to be thin. I don't want any of this stuff as much as I want to be thin." Over and over again. Every time I'd push my little shopping cart into a department with pastry, cookies, candy, snacks, I'd concentrate on "thin" and repeat the words in my mind: "I don't want it—I want to be thin!"

It may sound silly, but it worked! And from now on, every time I'm anywhere near high-calorie food, I'm putting my brain into remote repeat: "I don't want it. I want to be thin. I'm going to be thin. I will be thin. I'm getting thinner all the time!"

When I arrived home and unloaded my sack, I had those dangerous little packages of M&M's right in my hot little fingers. I forced myself to think it again: "I'm going to be thin!" Later, I thought of filling Jenny's gumball machine with M&M's for her secret pal. But, I'm proud to say, my mind reverberated with a resounding, "No! You feel safe right now, Rosemary. You feel strong. But if you open the package, it might be too tempting. So, no! Let Jenny fill the bank herself!" And so, I didn't swallow one little poison pill! I refused to take that last, dangerous step over the cliff. My feet were on firm ground with the bag of M&M's unopened. But who knows how far I'd have fallen if I had taken that stupid, last step. If I had lost my balance. If I had—gasp—opened the blasted bag.

Thursday, March 10, 1988
261 pounds

I feel wonderful. Eleven pounds to my next goalpost of 250. Oh, what a crazy life. To be so hypnotized by food. To be so totally consumed by consuming calories. It's bizarre. Compare it to your worst compelling behavior, your worst habit. Now stop the habit . . . forever! It ain't that easy, is it?

I want to be me again. I am tired of this boring, stay-at-home person who is mortified to go anywhere. I want to look up old friends. I crave their company. I want to know how they're doing. I miss them and would like to see them, but I'm so ashamed of myself, I'd rather die first. Janet Jones. Pam Torgrimson. Patti West. Karla Pjesky. Joan Clark. Peggy Davis. Bonnie Miller. Marilyn Larson. Where are you?

How are you? And your parents? I'm always wanting to stop by and see them, but I can't. I'm a double lardo. It would be embarrassing for all of us when they couldn't even recognize me!

Friday, March 11, 1988
260 pounds

A crazy thing happens when an overweight person honestly tries to diet. Suddenly *everyone* knows positively *everything* about what that person should or should not eat. Like yesterday, for instance. I was eating my breakfast: one small banana. I was feeling almost healthy, smug, and cute. A friend of mine was visiting. A fat friend of mine was visiting. A *very* fat friend of mine was visiting. This very fat friend gave her very free advice: "You know, you should stay away from bananas. They have a lot of natural sugars in them. Bananas, oranges, and apples all do."

Well, la-di-da-da. I wanted to stick out my tongue at her. I, a thirty-six-year-old woman, wanted to stick out my tongue and put a thumb in each of my ears and give her the raspberry! "Bananas have natural sugar"! Give me a break! You want to hear about sugar? How does my average breakfast grab you? One tuna sandwich, three cookies, and a handful of chips (while making school lunches for my children); a bowl of cereal and milk, and two pieces of buttered toast, generously sprinkled with cinnamon sugar (with the family, as they eat breakfast); a bowl of yogurt; half an orange; two more cookies (as I fix the baby's breakfast); two more pieces of buttered toast, lavishly covered with raspberry jam; two more cookies (as I make toast and milk for my husband to eat while he's dressing for work); five more cookies and a glass of milk for me as I sit and enjoy a few moments of uninterrupted eating. After all, I deserve a calm moment, and there is no such thing as sitting down to relax without food, is there?

Most of the above I stuffed into my mouth as I progressed

from one duty to the next. I wasn't even able to enjoy it. Cram and chew, cram and chew. Yup, that was my average breakfast. Just try and measure *that* sugar content! Then it's time to get the baby and the baby-sitting kids a snack . . . and you know what that means!

Yet this woman, this self-appointed adviser, thoughtlessly said, "You should stay away from bananas!" Bananas! Ha! Who ever heard of a fat monkey, for crying out loud?

Sunday, March 13, 1988
256 pounds

I've lost sixteen pounds in one week! I am full of hope. Allen and I had an important talk yesterday. He told me some things and expressed his feelings about my obesity that he had never before admitted. I cried and I laughed; I ached over what I had done to myself, to us. I longed for the experiences I've missed. I looked forward, as never before, to a new, skinny me.

Spring is in the air, and for the first time in years, I am looking forward to summer. Summer can be such a dreadful thing to think about. Who could possibly look forward to another fat summer? But not this year. I have three full months before summer vacation begins. With much dedicated effort, I can lose another fifty pounds by then. I've already lost sixteen pounds in one week! Of course, I can't continue to lose this fast all the way down to my ideal weight. But I need to get down to 199 quickly. I can live with being merely "fat"; it's this morbid obesity that drives me nuts and severely limits my activities and fun.

Wednesday, March 16, 1988
255 pounds

Last night I went freako. For no valid reason, I was uncontrol-lably angry at all the children. Allen and I came home from a church meeting at 9:15. Before I left, I had told the children to do their responsibilities and get to bed. But here was Jenny helping Tiffany write in her journal. Allen was impressed with the sweetness of the moment they were sharing. But I saw only the negative: Tiff wasn't in bed, Tyler was asleep on the front-room floor, and Jeremy hadn't put the diapers in the drier when he should have. I blew a gasket.

I am mortified. I don't even want to talk about it, to apolo-gize for it. I hope if I don't mention it, it will be forgotten, and I can crawl away and pretend the whole miserable night out of my life.

It's awful to be that out of control. I cannot describe my shame. Tuesday morning I was furious again, this time with Matthew. It was a buildup of lots of dumb-kid things. I screamed in his face. I told him I was packing his bags and sending him away that very night. Oh, dear God, can you ever forgive me for that? I can hardly write this. I want desperately to go back in time and change the whole morning, wipe out the whole hideous memory. It is a torture to live with. Can true repentance erase this horrible ache? And I slapped his face. Oh, dear little Matthew, what have I done?

I felt mean and rotten and horrible during both experiences. I knew I was out of control and ugly and wrong. Both times, I marched into the kitchen and ate like a pig. I *never* want to feel that way again. It is imperative that I lose weight and stop allowing my fat to be a catalyst for my temper. For then my temper becomes a catalyst for my fat.

Being fat is hell, but losing my temper with those I love is worse! The problem is, I know I won't *stop* losing my temper until I *start* losing my fat! I never again want to feel this ashamed. I never again want to have to record such a horrible memory of my own making. Writing about it is good punishment.

Wednesday, April 13, 1988
260 pounds

I don't know if I'm more crestfallen or more furious about my actions right now. Either way, I can hardly write today. Yes, I fell off. The minute I quit doing my workbook. I've gained back five pounds. The only thought that keeps me from going crazy is that I weigh twelve pounds less than I did five weeks ago.

It's hard to contemplate beginning a diet again. It's like purposely opening an old wound. It hurts! I feel like a soldier on a battlefield. I have been trampled over by the enemy, left for dead. I feel the life slowly oozing out of me; I am bleeding all over. It is extremely difficult to breathe. I wish I were dead, at last, and all would end.

Shakespeare knew exactly what I mean when he wrote, ''To be, or not to be. That is the question.'' Ah, yes, Hamlet's soliloquy was a marvelous example of how I feel: Is it worth it to go on living? Death may be the unknown, but surely it is better, or at least easier, than this present feeling of lying on the battlefield. Actually, it's not the lying on the ground in pain and misery that is so awful, it's the knowing that I have to get up.

The first day of dieting is like raising my head up a few inches. No one can imagine the agony. Yet tomorrow I must inflict more intense pain on myself as I struggle to lift my shoulders off the ground. In a week, I can be on my feet. But if I do get on my feet—and possibly take a few steps—will I ever be able to run? Or will I fall back down again?

My alleged ''buddy,'' Debbie, will help me for a few days and then get too busy and forget. She will do nothing for me unless *I* initiate it. I've been trying and trying. I have to soup myself up and then drag her with me. Well, this time I will lose ten pounds before I talk to Debbie about it, and if she doesn't want to come along with me, I'll do it myself. I'm not going to try to drag anyone anymore. It slows me down too much.

Allen, too, is of little help. Oh, I'm sure he *wants* to help, he wants me to be thin. You'd think a man would give his wife the daily fifteen minutes it takes to help her lose that saggy roll of fat that hangs between them every time they embrace. Especially when his wife begs for his help. I think if I were in bed with cancer, he would talk to me fifteen minutes a day. He would somehow make the time. If I were an alcoholic, he would devote himself to my recovery. Oh, but I *am* sick, depressed, and miserable to live with, so why won't he help me now? I'm screaming out for help!

> *January 11, 1992. As I read and reread my diary, I find myself shocked at the pain I feel from its pages. Life is so full of hope for me right now that I had forgotten much of the horror. I'm thankful for these recorded pages, so I may read and always remember—with a passion—that I never want to feel like that again! I know that it is no coincidence that when I am rereading my diary periodically, I lose weight.*

Friday, April 15, 1988
253 pounds

Three days! Three whole days. Seventy-two hours of being fantastic! The first day was sheer hell, as I recorded. The battlefield was real! It sounds absurd to say the enemy was chocolate bars, bread, pastries, cookies, and ice cream marching at me—all bearing my name, in neon lights, no less. Absurd—but true! I swear, every yummy treat in town chants a siren's song as I walk by it. But I beat them down. I shot them all full of holes. I didn't buy a single sweet thing.

I didn't whip up one chocolate-chip cookie or one cake. I won that battle and I'm standing tall. In fact, I feel like running.

Wednesday, April 27, 1988
248 pounds

Yikes! I am slipping. One day I even bought three candy bars. I wish I could say they tasted like rotten sawdust! But no, they were divine.

If I could do that once a week and then not bonk out, it would probably be good for me. But I'm afraid that since those fateful three bars, I've thought of chocolate even more. Then again, I haven't been doing my Daily Checklist.

I can feel my resolve dissolving. Here and now, I'm digging in my heels again. Onward and downward!

Tuesday, May 10, 1988
244 pounds

Back down to 244 today—whew! I will starve myself, if I have to, in order to be 199 by June 27—girls' camp. I want to go swimming while I'm there, and I refuse to be the fattest counselor in camp!

I'm beginning to feel the difference. I was recently washing my leg in the shower, and I realized, "Wow! My leg is smaller around. I can actually see less of it!" When I shut my eyes, I could *feel* less of it. I loved it. I'm also smaller across my shoulders. My clothes are hanging looser, and I can wear some clothes that had been too tight. I dream all day about what I am going to do and buy as the new and improved me!

Debbie was grouchy with me this morning. Some time ago, she officially asked me to be her "buddy." Trying to do my job today, I asked her how her maintenance plan was going. She became irrationally upset and snapped back, "Don't ask me that again!" Well, excuuuuse me! That's the last time—I mean the *very* last time—that she'll hear me ask that question. I will win this most difficult battle on my own. I am tired of being rebuffed.

Wednesday, May 11, 1988
243 pounds

Yesterday I was weeding in my flower garden, when I suddenly realized, "Hey! This is easier than the last time I weeded. I can bend over without hurting." You can't imagine how painful some body positions are for the fat person, both inside and out. When I'm on my knees, bending over to do yard work, it causes my lungs to become all squished inside, and it's hard to breathe. My fat rolls are pressed so hard into each other that they ache! It's possible to squish only a certain amount of fat into any given space. When I sit down and then bend over, the fat is especially compacted, and yowie! It hurts. How many roly-polies do you see doing yard work? Believe me, the brave ones who do are huffing and puffing and grunting away!

Anyway, I'm feeling and seeing differences in my body. Not only was it easier doing yard work yesterday, it's much simpler getting in and out of the Opel GT. Sports cars were not designed for obese people. And I can see a visible reduction in the width of my shoulders—yahoo! Forty-four more pounds, and I leave the realm of the obese forever. When I weigh 199, I will feel simply "fat." Ha! I am actually looking forward to being fat!

September 21, 1991. In the three years since I wrote that entry, I have read hundreds of articles about obesity. I am dreadfully sorry to have to write that at 199 pounds, I would still be obese. The clinical definition of obesity is 20 percent or more over your ideal body weight. If my perfect weight were 140 pounds, I would be obese at 169 pounds. Gee whiz! A paltry 169 sounds nearly emaciated to me right now!

Friday, May 13, 1988
241 pounds

I *love* to think thin. Have I ever completely explained what it is? I usually think thin while stretched out on my bed. I shut my eyes and I remember. I think back. I recall specific times in my life when I was thin and alluring. I relive the moment. I mentally enter that thin body and exult in its freedom of movement. I jump and dance and run and play and stand in a sexy pose or two. I *become* thin . . . for a time. Then I open my workbook to my Weight-Loss Goal Calendar. I study and plan and thrill over each day, each page. I mentally visualize myself at each stage of weight loss.

At 225, I will fit into three more dresses. I can hardly wait to have a choice again. Twenty-one more pounds, and I will ride my bike again. I will weigh a disgusting 220 pounds, but I will then have the courage to haul my hulk onto my bike and enjoy freedom of movement again. I never in a million years would have thought that one day, at age thirty-five, I would be dying to ride my bike.

Tuesday, May 24, 1988
238 pounds

I am officially through with Debbie as a buddy! We had committed to exercise together and encourage each other on our diets. I called her this morning to report on my success: "I've lost ten pounds since you last saw me! Can we get together to exercise today?" I was stunned by her response:

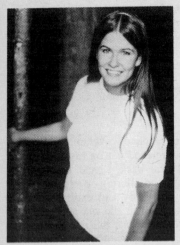
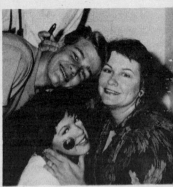

August 1970, 130 pounds, and November 1987, 250 pounds. While thinking thin, I visualize my "sweater girl" days, not my "sweaty girl" days. Here I weigh more than Jennifer and Jeremy combined!

"Oh, heavens, no!" I held in my hurt and disappointment. Gee, Debbie, I'm elated over this additional ten-pound loss. I needed to hear some words of praise, a simple, "Rose, that's great! But sorry—I'm too busy to exercise today."

When I asked her about tomorrow, she replied she was too busy then, also. She had to pack for a trip that was three days away. Good grief, it takes only half an hour to exercise! So I asked, "When *can* we get together?" Debbie rather angrily retorted, "Next Tuesday!" Next Tuesday is a whole week away! Next Tuesday, my eye! You'll undoubtedly pick up a few pounds on your vacation, Debbie. And the way I feel right now, that will be just fine with me!

Learn from my experience: Pick your buddy carefully!

Wednesday, June 15, 1988
240 pounds

If I lose fifteen pounds before girls' camp, I will weigh 225. I'm afraid my camp-goal of 199 is forever lost to me. What a tragedy. I'll be too fat to go swimming. I won't even be able to climb a hill without huffing and puffing. I've done it to myself and my family again—another *fat* summer.

> *February 7, 1991. I did go to girls' camp. I did not, however, weigh 225 or less. But even at that, I wasn't the fattest counselor there! Remember my church meeting where I count all the fat ladies? I think half of them also volunteered to be counselors at camp.*

Monday, June 20, 1988
? pounds

Five days later, and I am definitely feeling suicidal. I am out of control. I am eating *everything* I see. We hosted a wedding reception for my niece last night. We inherited all the leftovers, and I have stuffed everything I could see, touch, or smell into my mouth for the last twenty-four hours. I'm sure I've gained at least five pounds.

I don't want to weigh myself. I'm terrified of weighing myself. If I climb back up the hell scale, I will die. I'm sure I will. Yet who am I kidding? At 240 pounds, I've already climbed mighty high up that miserable, fat-measuring device. I've been having chest pains again. It scares me to death. Yesterday my knees felt all swollen and stiff. What I am doing to my body is as cruel as it is absurd. I wouldn't dream of asking my husband to carry a 100-pound sack of flour from one room to the next. Yet I ask my poor joints to suffer under that load, and much more, every second of every day.

But it's not over till the fat lady sings, and I will yet be somebody . . . besides the fat lady!

Debbie may be moody and undependable as a buddy, but she and I still have some good laughs together. Yesterday we delved into our bizarre childhood eating habits and our almost desperate love of ice cream. We ate gallons of it every summer during our youth.

My dad loved ice cream. But then, what decent human being doesn't? Living close to an Albertsons store, we drove past it often. We could purchase a double-scoop cone for the incredibly low price of one shiny nickel! It was a good deal, even back then. In the summer months, my dad would often stop and buy us all a double-scoop cone.

There was nothing wrong with buying us an ice cream cone—not the first one. The problem arose when Dad would announce that anyone who finished his or her cone by the time we drove to the next ice cream store would get a second cone. Because the next store was only a few blocks away, we kids almost choked down those first cones, not enjoying a single bite. We swallowed them so fast that we had headaches from the cold. We pounded our foreheads with the palms of our hands to try to alleviate the sudden, intense pain. And why? To qualify for our second double-scoop cone in five minutes! It was pathetic. We ate too much, too fast. We were rewarded for being little pigs.

Even in placing the order for the cone, we learned we had to act fast or lose our chance. My dad wasn't exactly known for his patience. When the lady behind the counter asked what flavor we wanted, we practically had to spit it out at her. If we hesitated one second too long, we went without!

It wasn't until I became a mother myself that I realized what a pleasure it is for parents to give treats to their children. And, of course, to themselves. I am now all too aware that my parents bought treats for themselves every bit as much as they did "for the children." Believe me, I know the tricks parents pull to get their sweet tooth satisfied. Many, many times I have purchased "treats for the kids" that were earmarked expressly for me!

My parents didn't realize that they were establishing a lifetime of horrible eating habits for their children. Thirty years ago, the term *eating disorder* was unheard of. And besides, we children were all very active and thin. The "Lind kids" were the recognized athletes at Harvey Scott Grade School. Our own backyard was a virtual park. We played kick-the-can, tag, dare-base, hide-and-seek. If we had been like the TV-watching, video game–playing kids of today, we might have had weight problems as children. But it wasn't until my siblings and I became adults that those old pounds started acting up! (Or should I say "adding up"?)

I think it's important for me to recognize the roots of my eating disorder. A popular therapy of today is to dig into one's childhood to find the source of one's dysfunctional behaviors. (In fact, it seems to me that we look more for causes than for cures.) Okay, so now I've dug. I have this huge pile of dirt by my side. I recognize the error of many of my childhood ways. But, that accomplished, why do I still want a pound—and a half—of chocolate malt balls?

Saturday, July 9, 1988
248 pounds

I am writing now on the verge of tears. On the verge of screaming. Perhaps, on the verge of—dare I write it again?— suicide. I am totally miserable. The last two days I have lost myself in reading. I desperately want to find happiness, to find the key to self-control. I try to find some escape in my silly little novels, living the fascinating life of the heroine.

I feel silly admitting that I am reading *Tarzan of the Apes*, but I am and I love it. I fantasize about being carried through the trees by the strongest, most handsome man in the world. But always the awful reality hits me: even Tarzan couldn't carry me through the jungle. Nor would he ever want to. (At my present weight, Tarzan would have a hard time carrying me in *water*!) How I long to be thought lovely and feminine again. How I long for my freedom from this hell-cell. How I crave my once graceful body again, unfettered by 400 sticks of butter.

I am depressed and hateful of myself because I have once again ruined another summer. Jeremy asked if our family could go on the Alpine Slide. Oh, sure! All 248 pounds of me. I cannot write of the horror I fear that awaits me if I don't stop this hideous eating. Life has become less than useless.

Thursday, July 21, 1988
246 pounds

Yesterday was my uncle Chuck Ball's funeral. His family asked Allen and me to be the speakers. I am not good at funerals. I hate getting so emotional in front of everyone. I get embarrassed, but I can't help it. I was thankful that while giving the eulogy, I was able to control my tears. I enjoyed writing it. I felt especially close to Uncle Chuck while researching his life. I feel empty when I think that Uncle Chuck's earthly life is over. He was always nice to me. I enjoyed his sense of humor, his stories, and especially his beautiful singing voice. I will miss him.

The whole experience abruptly reminded me of the shortness of life. The swiftness with which one can leave this frail existence. Funerals are also times of great recommitment for me. So I sat crying at his funeral, determined to make more of myself. Determined to be kinder, to show more patience, to do all the nice things I desire to do for those I love. Determined to get organized, so I can take advantage of every minute of the life I have left. Even determined to lose weight, so I can more fully enjoy this sensational world, so I can become a participant in life again.

After the funeral, Chuck's sister had the family over to her home for a meal. Everything looked delicious. Desserts were in abundance. When I saw them displayed there in all their glory, my eyes nearly bulged out of my head. I could almost hear the *beep, beep, beep—red alert, red alert* from *Star Trek*. My palms started to sweat. I grabbed Allen so fast I almost gave him whiplash. I immediately whispered in his ear, before I had a second to change my mind, "I'm not having *any* desserts or punch." There! I said it. I committed to someone *before* temptation was able to suck me in and swallow me whole. I could breathe easier now. I'd be okay. I'd made a commitment.

I dished up my plate once, ate slowly, and stopped. The single thing I had seconds of was water! I ate a wafer-thin slice of turkey and one of ham, three slices of tomato, and some fresh fruit. I won that round.

I keep hearing that song in my head: "This time we almost made it, didn't we, girl?" Only, I sing, "This time I'm gonna make it! I'm gonna be thin! This time you're gonna make it, girl!"

Friday, July 29, 1988
240 pounds

I recently read a wonderful article in *Towers Club USA Newsletter*. It stated a plain and simple truth. We each have twenty-four hours given to us every day. Twenty-four golden hours. In this, we *are* created equal. The author of the article compared these hours to money. We can use the money daily, but we can't accumulate it. Once the day is over, our money is gone, whether we use it or not. Some people make worthwhile investments with their "money." Others do nothing. It is up to us to use it wisely or lose it completely.

This article, although simple, had a tremendous impact on me. It's true. We all *do* have the same twenty-four hours given to us. Have I used my hours wisely? I am distressed with what I must admit. I fritter away my time, my very life, on many worthless things. Television is at the top of the list. That life-sucking box on my shelf, that hypnotizing little cube that often fills my mind with filthy words and trashy deeds and less than noble actions.

Although I firmly believe in reading good books (we have a library in our home with thousands of books), insignificant books are a dreadful waste of time. For the last couple of years, I have tried to stick to classic literature—uplifting, educational, inspiring works. When I recently finished *To Kill a Mockingbird*, I felt almost reverent, as though I had experienced a sacred moment. I thought to myself, "I have touched minds and spirits with a noble person."

I have several other insane, unproductive habits. The next in line is that I flit. I start to clean the kitchen. I take a brush off the drainboard to put in the bathroom. While in the bathroom, I proceed to start straightening it, which leads me to my bedroom, the utility room, the garage, the attic. Suddenly the day is over, and not one visible task has been accomplished. Nothing! I've "flitted" all day from room to room, and nothing looks much better. *But* . . . ray of sunshine! There is hope. I analyzed my behavior and have come up with a solution. If an item doesn't belong in the room I'm trying to clean, I put it in a box. Then, when I'm through in that room, I empty the box and put everything where it belongs. It works! My flitting days are over.

Another serious problem *was* my acute "grazing" tendency. All day long I would find myself in the kitchen, wondering what there was to eat. In reality, I knew full well: there was exactly the same thing to eat as there was ten-fifteen-thirty minutes ago. But I'd recheck the fridge, the freezer, the cupboards anyway. Maybe twenty times a day.

For almost two weeks, I haven't grazed once. Each morning, I decide what I will eat that day; then I write it down. I don't sit around and dream about food. Eating has become a necessary inconvenience. I wish it were possible to stop eating completely. I could stop worrying about food altogether. I find myself saying, "I have to eat something. I really must keep my strength up." Ha! *That* is a miraculous change of attitude. And think of all the time I now save. At least three hours a day. That's way more time than it takes to do my Daily Checklist. Significant discovery! Doing my checklist doesn't *take* time . . . it *makes* time!

Saturday, July 30, 1988
240 pounds

Last week, I accompanied Allen to a church dance where he was playing the drums. There I saw one of my friends, Deanna DeLong. She always makes me feel good. As if I'm someone special. As if I am a remarkably talented person! We talked for nearly two hours about the jillion and one things that had happened in our lives since we had last seen one another. I told her how proud—and envious—I was of her impressive accomplishments. Then she restated what I had read in that Towers Club publication only days before: "Rosemary, we all have the same twenty-four hours in a day. I make conscious efforts each day to do certain things. Like running. Probably three days a week, I have to make myself get up at four-thirty A.M. I'd rather sleep longer. But it's up to me to succeed. It's my choice."

I've repeated those words a lot lately: "We all have the same twenty-four hours in a day. It is up to me to succeed. It's my choice." And here's one girl who's going to make her twenty-four hours count. Each day . . . *every* day!

Monday, August 1, 1988
239 pounds

Men are chauvinists. For the most part, men have always expected women to "do" for them. After church yesterday, Allen disappeared into his room and took a nap. He didn't tell me where he was going. He just expected someone to wake him up when dinner was ready. I have five children to take care of and a meal to fix. What did he think I should do? Follow him around and take note of where he decided to relax? Well, I didn't, so no one knew where he was when we sat down for dinner. And get this! When he did get up, he became angry at me and said how awful I was. Why? Because I asked him to let me know in the future when he was going to take naps while I fixed his dinner. "Oh, yes, my Lord. It's done, my Lord. Would you like it in bed, my Lord? Can I get you something else, my Lord?"

It was Sunday, for crying out loud! We were *both* commanded to rest on the Sabbath. Why should I cook while he sleeps? Chauvinism! It isn't fair! Now, if he had told me he was so tired he was sick, I would have said, "Poor baby . . . go take a nap! What time do you want to get up for dinner?" But please, show me a little respect.

That was only one event from yesterday. Everything else was as bad or worse. It ended by my telling my children and husband that I wished I'd never married or had children. It was partly true. I am so sick and tired of feeling like a failure that it seems it would have been better never to have tried.

Wednesday, August 3, 1988
236 pounds

It is an adventure as I daily discover new, "thinner" parts of me. I was sitting on my bed yesterday with one leg curled up under me. (Doesn't that sound almost petite and sexy, conjuring up an image of a delicate nymph with red-polished toenails?) I noticed that my knee was smaller. I could feel the bones and see a little shape. I was excited because it didn't look like a beach ball with a dent in it.

Allen's thirty-year high school reunion is in ten days. I want to take advantage of those ten days and lose 100 pounds. Okay, I would be thrilled to lose ten. I want it for Allen as much as for me.

Oh, please, life, wait for me. A few more months, and I will be able to join in with you again. I am full of hope and anticipation. I cannot begin to comprehend how I could ever let a candy bar change it all to absolute misery and despair. I need my daily "upper," my Daily Checklist. It keeps me higher than a kite, and it's cheaper than doing drugs. It is healthy and safe and uplifting.

Thursday, August 4, 1988
232 pounds

I am angry with myself. Several reasons. First, I let people manipulate me. I hate myself for it. I'm constantly bombarded by daily phone calls from people who need to talk over their problems. I innocently pick up the phone, then suddenly it is two hours later, and I have done nothing on my checklist. I have to protect myself from being inadvertently drawn into other people's problems. At present, it is critical that I start putting my own screwed-up life in order. I need to turn on my answering machine more often.

Today Mom called. She was feeling depressed. She offered to take me out to lunch. (Yes, that is the mentality I grew up with: If you're depressed, eat your blues away.) Knowing I couldn't afford the calories, I bravely said no. But I was moved by the need to do something to lift her out of her doldrums, so I suggested she come with me to run some errands.

True to form with my family, she requested that our last stop be a drive-through restaurant. We picked up some food and drove to Debbie's house, where I (oh, I am so proud) ate nothing. The whole time I was with them, I knew there were more important things I needed to be doing than to sit there and watch them eat. Starting today, I must avoid interruptions till I've completed my Daily Checklist. I must start putting me first!

I'm also angry with myself because I ate too much food last night. I went to a potluck dinner. Need I say more? I foolishly allowed my own pan of warm zucchini bread to stay parked right in front of me. I was defenseless sitting near it. It jumped into my mouth. I wish I'd had the courage to move that bread away from me. I wish at least one member of my family had loved me enough to do so.

Monday, August 15, 1988
228 pounds

Last night I bonked. I was in my bedroom, thinking of my list, realizing I hadn't done it for three days, and . . . *zap*! I ran down the hall to the kitchen and shoved a big bite of frosting into my mouth. Fortunately, I stopped there. But it scared me.

As I walked back to my room, I felt like a bad dog slinking down the hallway with its tail tucked between its legs. I felt slimy and low and disgusting. I resolved then and there to do my list today. I never want to feel like a bad dog again.

I don't want to go out to dinner anymore without first discussing it with Allen. I was fairly good both Friday and Saturday nights. But it's impossible to eat as few calories when I dine out as when I eat a frozen, packaged, low-calorie meal. I need to be super careful of where we eat out and then stay committed to eating small portions. It's essential to bring my own low-calorie dressing for the salad and butter-flavored seasoning for the potato. I used to use at least one-and-a-half tablespoons of dressing on my salad and one-and-a-half tablespoons of butter on my potato. That's 300 calories of pure fat. Yikes! That's more calories than in a frozen meal!

There seems to be something almost magical about frozen meals. They are self-contained in one tidy package. No snitching. I eat only what's in the tray. If I eat it slowly and concentrate on the fact that it is my whole dinner, then it is enough. It is delicious and satisfying. I love them!

Frozen meals are perfect for me. I can't fix two different dinners each day—one for the family, one for me. I prepare one meal for the family and pop one frozen dinner into the microwave for me. What could be simpler? An added delight is that I don't have to worry about what the family is eating. I don't have to consider their calorie count. I can fix them anything. Their meal simply doesn't exist for me. I don't taste it, I just serve it. My frozen meals seem to have the magical quality of insulating me from the temptation to eat any other foods. When I sit down to my own little frozen meal, I feel like a queen! The children always say how yummy it smells and how delicious it looks. Occasionally, I'll give one of them a bite of something, but usually I savor every morsel for myself . . . and feel good about it.

Friday, August 19, 1988
228 pounds

I was at one of Jeremy's softball games last night. Jennifer told me she was looking at some women standing around talking, when she noticed that one lady had skinny legs. "Then I looked up at the person—and it was you, Mom!" Yessss!

Sunday, September 18, 1988
232 pounds

I can't believe that I have been off my diet for a full month. I was on like a rock for a month. I looked forward to all the things I could do when I was thin. I was up and cheerful and encouraging to be around, and I want to be that way again!

Lately, I have been completely depressed, but I have been putting up a pretty good front. But inside I am feeling the constant terror of climbing back up the hell scale. I feel unusually huge. Though I am down a full forty pounds, I feel bigger than I ever have.

Today I weigh 232, but tomorrow it will be 230 or less. Two weeks from today, I will break my own "pound barrier" of 216 and be down a full 57 pounds. I will weigh only 215.

A mere five pounds more, and I will try on all my clothes again to see what new, smaller items I will then be able to wear.

> *July 23, 1991. It makes me laugh as I read all the little details of "how many pounds I must lose to reach such-and-such a point." It sounds ridiculous. Yet, to the dieter, those details are critically important. In fact, show me a dieter who isn't preoccupied with numbers of pounds, days, and sizes, and I will show you a dieter who isn't dieting!*

Wednesday, September 28, 1988
233 pounds

I am fed up with myself! Ha! Fed up! Yup, that's me. I've been feeding myself up for over a month again. Each day, I think about doing my Daily Checklist, but I don't . . . and so I eat. And I hate myself! I'm sick and tired of it. In fact, that's more true than I care to admit. I *am* sick and tired. Almost every day for the last month, I have had stomachaches. Extreme nausea from eating pure garbage all day. Candy bars up the gazoo and with us so broke I can't afford groceries. Candy, ice cream, homemade birthday cakes, other sugary sweets—oh, yuck.

I am extremely nauseated by evening. I have gas pains in my chest. I am plagued by "rotten egg" burps. I hear and feel my stomach churning and rumbling. I have horrible gas and diarrhea. My body is warning me to *quit*. With all those problems, do you think I can sleep well? Heavens, no! Most of them occur at night! I lie there wide awake, feeling like I might die—hoping I will die. I want out of this pit of despair.

Tuesday, October 4, 1988
236 pounds

I must mean business today! I unabashedly asked Allen to lock up the stupid, dumb, horrible, ugly, fat-producing, diet-destroying, dream-wrecking, life-ruining candy bars he had "hidden" in his office. He's a sweet man, but he is a miserable failure as a candy-bar hider. In a sack by the side of his couch! Oh, brother!

I was walking down the hall to my bedroom one day when suddenly I was inspired by . . . hmmmm . . . let me think. Could it be Satan? Yes! I'd swear that Satan himself inspired me to remember Allen's comment from last night: "I bought some candy bars instead of cards to give as birthday greetings to my church class." Candy bars! I didn't care who or what they were for. Candy bars! I could always buy more to replace whatever I cleverly stole from Allen's supply today. Candy bars! I did an immediate U-turn on a dime, raced down the stairs to his office, took a full three seconds to look over the room for possible hiding places, and headed straight for the sack by the side of his couch, and *voilà*! Talk about being guided! Talk about sixth sense. Talk about cramming a candy bar in my mouth.

That kind of behavior has kept me fat for sixteen long years. So one more time. No, let's make that one *last* time: "I am fighting for my husband, my children, my freedom, my God, but most importantly right now—for me." So I have lost a few previous skirmishes. This time I shall win the war! "This time you're gonna make it, girl!"

Monday, October 17, 1988
228 pounds

I weigh 228 this morning. I'm not as low as I should be, but at least I'm on a downtrend. It's nice that there is one area in my life where being down makes me feel up. I want to feel elated again. I want to be excited about new clothes, about Christmas, about this winter, about next summer! And right now, I want a coat that will button around me!

Same day, 4:08 P.M.
228 pounds

I am making this entry in absolute desperation. I mean, I am ready to claw the skin off my face for a candy bar, yet I would give up ten years of my life to be thin! I want to be sexy. I want to be free. I want to be happy.

This is the worst time of day for me. From about 3:00 to 5:00 P.M. I feel like one of those huge whales that glide through the ocean with their cavernous mouths hanging open. I suck in everything edible. Yup, I eat like a whale . . . and I look like a whale. It's horrible!

I have to go buy a head of lettuce for dinner. How those words send a shiver of fear down my spine. "I have to go buy ———." Don't you understand? I'll be in a store. *In a store, do you hear me?* I'll be near cookies, pastry, candy, ice cream. I will want to buy them all. My cart will make a beeline—almost as if on train tracks—to those departments. I will have to clamp my jaws shut tightly. I will have to wipe my sweaty palms on my sides so that I will be able to keep control of the cart. I will have to hush up some 500 billion fat cells that are screaming out to be nourished. I will have to somehow pull away from the intense magnet that draws me ever back to gaze, with longing eyes and quivering lips, at the beautifully wrapped candy bars. This is not some slight wish or mild craving. I go *crazy* for candy bars! I lust after them, okay? And once I pull in my stomach and suck in my cheeks and stand especially tall and draw up my double chin and readjust all my clothes to appear as thin as possible while waiting in line to buy the candy bars, no one will ever know I bought them, right?

Tuesday, October 25, 1988
232 pounds

I had a horrible day yesterday! My brother Mark came to our house . . . drunk again. "That demon rum" has poor Mark by the throat. While I have spent the last sixteen years of my life eating myself into an out-of-control piggo, he has spent those same years in various stages of inebriation. Allen and I have tried desperately to help Mark. Alcoholism is a horrible disease, difficult for the drinker *and* his family to cope with. I am only beginning to learn how to deal with it.

I'm afraid we made the situation worse by being "enablers" for the past ten years, providing my brother a place to crash after many of his big drunks. Allen and I have finally realized our innocent mistake. We point-blank told Mark, "Get out. Get out and never come back. You cannot live here anymore. You are thirty-one years old and have the ability to take care of yourself! Go to your AA meetings, but don't come here anymore!"

Well, Mark came yesterday, drunker than a skunk! (Has anyone ever really seen a drunk skunk?) He was rude. He was obnoxious. He scared me. He threatened to call the police because I pushed him out of my yard. He screamed out horrible, vile words in the street.

There he was, screaming at the top of his lungs in our front yard, and all we had ever done to Mark was offer him assistance. Cook him food. Help dry him out. Take him to detox centers. Pick him up at taverns at three o'clock in the morning. Wash his clothes. Give him haircuts. Listen to his woes. Invite him in for holidays. Be "Santa" to him. I—who have never touched a cigarette in my life and am adamantly opposed to the filthy habit—I even drove him to the store *many* times and gave him money to buy cigarettes! (The cigarettes seemed a mild addiction when compared to the alcohol and helped Mark stay sane.)

I cried all afternoon. I was so frustrated. I kept asking, "Why, God? Why do you allow Mark to turn my life upside-down this way? Why, when I am merely trying to help him, does it seem to backfire so terribly?'' (I just answered the phone, and it was Mark, calling to apologize, even as I was writing about him in my diary!)

Anyway, that all happened yesterday. Of course, this morning the incident was heavy on my mind. As I was mulling over my anger and feeling sorry for myself, I suddenly became aware of an analogy between Mark and me. Mark drinks out of control, an alcoholic desperate to stop. I am a ''foodaholic'' who is also desperate to stop. The next time I reach for a cookie, a sandwich, a candy bar, or ice cream, I must remember Mark. Think of Mark. Concentrate on Mark. My addiction, though not alcohol, is similarly devastating my life, sucking up my freedom and happiness, ruining all I might become. I am as out of control as he is. I must never forget Mark. Maybe that's God's answer to my Why? after all.

> *September 25, 1991. It is splendid to be able to acknowledge that Mark has been dry for about a year and a half. His struggle to overcome has been an inspiration to me. Although alcoholism is a hideous disease, I can't help feeling a little jealous of his situation. We have both struggled with addictive disorders these long years. But Mark was dry the day after he quit drinking. Even after months of dieting, I am still fat.*

Wednesday, November 2, 1988
226 pounds

I want out of here! Away from blubber! Removed from fat! I am committed today. I've prayed for help, and now I'm going to do all that I can to earn it.

Number one thing is to have Allen lock up all the Halloween candy. Don't laugh. I'm serious! If it's locked up in a suitcase, it's almost as if it's not there. I don't find myself wandering in every five minutes to see which yummy little morsel I can devour, what "fun size" bar I can discover. I don't have to ask myself which of my children's bags of goodies I can shake up, fluff up enough, to hide the fact that I took more out. No, it's locked up. It's not there. I can't get it. I don't think about it. Except for maybe . . . I find myself shaping old bobby pins into cute little . . . suitcase-type keys.

Tuesday, January 10, 1989
241 pounds

Sixty-nine days since an entry. Thanksgiving and Christmas and New Year's without an entry. *And*, without an entry, fifteen more pounds of me! Ayeeee!

Have you ever seen a scary movie where the heroine is chased by some raving maniac with a knife? Running frantically, she becomes exhausted, then—horrid twist of fate—finds herself in a room with only one doorway. The maniac is mere seconds behind her. Instinctively, she dashes, screaming hysterically, to the far corner, only to turn and face her relentless attacker. There is nowhere to go, no escape, no way out. What a terrifying prospect. What a hideous thought. Yet I live that feeling every day.

I am in constant terror as I experience the feeling of being out of control. Where can I go? What will I do? Doesn't anyone understand? I am getting fatter by the day. I hate myself for each bite; I detest my reflection, but I can't stop shoveling food into my mouth. There is nowhere to go, no escape, no way out. I'm in the corner with the raving maniac lunging toward me. I accidentally touch a hidden switch, and an impenetrable shield drops down to protect me. No, like a beam of light from above, my workbook appears before me. I only have to touch it to feel a magical calm, an intense hope, a sense of comfort . . . a way to escape.

Thursday, January 12, 1989
238 pounds

I feel as if I'm walking on eggshells. I'm ecstatic with hope for the future and, at the same time, afraid to look ahead. I feel sure I'll make it this time. Yet twice before, I lost over fifty pounds and then somehow strayed from my diet. More often, I stray big time after only a few days.

I'm trying to protect myself, not being too sure or cocky. Keeping a continual prayer in my heart. Being strict on using my Daily Checklist. I'm thirty-six. I have to do it this time, or there might not be any more times to try. My obesity might finally do me in. If I don't shoot myself over my misery, I could die of heart failure. Think of my poor little heart, struggling doubly hard to keep two of me alive. Yesterday, I read an amazing fact in an anatomy book. For each pound a person is overweight, the body produces an estimated 200 miles of extra capillaries. Two hundred miles of teeny, tiny blood vessels. Do you know what that adds up to for me? Well, let's assume I am a paltry 125 pounds overweight. That is 25,000 miles of extra vessels through which my poor heart must pump blood. Good grief! That is the circumference of the earth, enough extra vessels to encircle the entire globe! No wonder fat people have a greater incidence of high blood pressure and strokes!

I want to be thin. I say it a hundred times a day! I want to be thin. I want to be pretty! I want it more than anything right now. More than a cookie or a candy bar, a sandwich or ice cream, or . . . any possible concoction I can put into my mouth!

Actually, I am quite good at concoctions. When I was growing up, I had to be. When the undeniable lust for something sweet hit, there was never anything sweet in my house to eat. Hence, I concocted!

This story cannot possibly be as funny in the telling as it was in the living, but Debbie and I get nearly hysterical every time we talk about it. I was about twelve years old, Debbie about eleven. We had just walked into the house from school. No one was home, which was very unusual. We were both hungry, which was not very unusual. The same thought entered both our minds at the same moment: What sweet thing was there to eat? Nothing in the cookie jar. We never had any sweets in our house. Sweets were systematically unwrapped and disposed of within seconds of entering the Lind atmosphere. So what were we to do?

We frantically searched the cupboards. No loose chocolate chip. No stale cookie. No dried-up ice cream sticking to the sides of the empty ice cream container. We were crazy for something sweet! Ah. We could make frosting, chocolate frosting. But we had to hurry because Mom's friend was coming momentarily to pick us up for a church class. We kept a sharp eye out the window in her direction.

Debbie grabbed half the ingredients; I snatched the rest. As I dumped some powdered sugar into a bowl, I asked, "Is she coming?"

"No! Hurry!"

I didn't bother measuring; just wanted that sugary, chocolaty stuff whipped together. I added the butter and vanilla. "Can you see her yet?"

Debbie, with a quick glance out the window: "No, can't you go any faster?"

Now it needed only a little milk and cocoa. I repeated with fresh intensity, "Is she coming?"

Debbie once again peered out the window in the direction from which our ride would arrive. "No."

Hooooonk!

Yikes! Somehow, we hadn't paid close enough attention. Our intense concentration on getting that chocolate frosting down our throats had backfired. We were stuck with half-done frosting, a mess on the kitchen counter, and a ride honking for us. What's a kid to do? We made our decision in an instant. We grabbed every trace of frosting and shoved the whole mess under our bed. Debbie ran out to the car while I ran a washcloth over the counter to erase any trace of our aborted attempt at culinary magic.

I'm not sure what we did with that half-made frosting under the bed. In order to finish mixing it up—without getting into trouble for making it in the first place—we would have had to be alone in the house. And that seldom happened. I can't believe that we threw it away. But I hope we did. It makes me feel good to think that somewhere out there is some chocolate that escaped my lips . . . my hips.

Saturday, January 14, 1989
238 pounds

I am in control. I am able to put things in perspective. When I'm near fattening foods, I purposely fill my brain full of thin thoughts: of soon being on a glorious business trip—alone with my husband—to Palm Springs; of skinniness; of prettiness; of new and fun activities. But first, I have to pay the price. It isn't enough to merely give up M&M's. Although that might be hell in itself, I have to do more. I have to pay the price for the billions of M&M's I've consumed in the past.

It's like repentance. To truly repent, there must be a restitution, if possible. The thief has the relatively simple task of repaying those from whom he stole, but the repentant fat person must literally give up part of herself. She must reduce her caloric intake to such a level that it compensates for all the pig-outs of the past. And that task cannot be done overnight. It is accomplished day by day, week by week, and month by month. Slowly making restitution to one's own body. Repenting to self, to mate, to family, to God. As slowly as the fat dissolves, the restitution is made. Eventually I will stand before a full-length mirror and proclaim to myself, "There! I paid you back. I am no longer in debt to you . . . to me. I am free."

Wednesday, January 18, 1989
232 pounds

Eight more measly pounds to reach my lowest weight in three years. I love being in control. I don't want to eat. I keep thin thoughts in my brain all day long. Palm Springs—I'll be thinner! Rose Festival—I'll look decent! Playing, going, doing—oh, yes! I don't even *want* that cookie. (Oh, wait . . . did you say it was an Otis Spunkmeyer brand chocolate-chip cookie? Just kidding!)

I have been furious with Allen and frantic out of my mind with Matt this last week, but *I did not eat*! I did not allow my emotions to let me explode into a frenzied eating fit. I controlled my thoughts. It takes thoughts to make actions, and only actions can make me fat. Only by putting the food into my mouth will I get fatter. If I control the thoughts, my actions *have* to follow!

Sunday, January 22, 1989
232 pounds

I have been incredibly busy with Matthew, trying to help him finish his schoolwork before the end of the semester. We stayed up until after midnight on Tuesday, Wednesday, and Thursday. Two and a half days without doing my workbook, and I was starting to stray. When I went grocery shopping last night, I almost committed the unpardonable sin: I almost bought a candy bar. I still want one. This is so darn hard. I need to remember the strength that I get from using my workbook. How can I possibly get too busy to fill it in each day? When will I learn to take care of me first?

Monday, January 23, 1989
232 pounds

I tore up my entry of January 15, 1989. I broke my own rule and wrote when I was mad. Mad is not the right word. I was furious. I was livid with rage. It was a mean, dumb entry, and I knew when I wrote it that I would destroy it later.

There was one part I thought was kind of funny, though. Quoting an ancient prophet, I wrote, "Men are that they might have joy." Then I injected the following insight: "Ha! That's probably the whole trouble. Man was meant to have joy . . . and woman was meant to go through agony to see that he achieved it." My final sentence in that masterpiece of meanness was important: "I'm not going off my diet over this." Isn't that astonishing? Livid with rage, but sticking to my diet.

Tuesday, January 24, 1989
232 pounds

I have been making every calorie count. You'd be amazed at how much you can consume and still stay under 800 calories a day. Yesterday I ate:

Breakfast:	One cup dry cereal	110 calories
	One banana	80 calories
Lunch:	One cup green beans	31 calories
	One-fourth cup tomato sauce	20 calories
	One chicken leg	90 calories
Dinner:	One chicken leg	90 calories
	One egg	80 calories
	One tomato	30 calories
	Two cups lettuce	10 calories
	One slice French bread	80 calories

	Four tablespoons lo-calorie dressing	16 calories
Snacks:	One pickle	7 calories
	One apple	80 calories
	One cup chicken broth	16 calories
	Two cups Sugar Free Jell-O	32 calories
		772 calories

I could have had three more pickles or two saltine crackers or all the lettuce or green peppers I wanted. There is no magic to 800 calories a day. I am aware that a diet of less than 800 calories is considered "too restrictive" and should be done only under a doctor's supervision. Let's be honest, I just listed a lot of food. And you don't have to cut back to 800 calories a day to lose weight. Many diets include 1,200 calories a day. That means you can eat half again as much food as I just listed . . . or a piddling three ounces of chocolate candy! When you see it in black and white, it seems unbelievable that we fatties ever choose the dumb candy.

Mark has been on a big drunk again. He is trying desperately to kick this alcohol addiction, but he never will until he's honest with himself. He won't accept the facts. He won't admit that his own lifestyle inevitably throws him back into alcohol every time he dries out. When he is sober, he doesn't look for work or take proper care of his personal hygiene. He doesn't shave or keep his room clean. He won't divorce himself from his old friends who encourage him to "have just one more!" Thus, being less than squeaky clean and surrounded by fellow drinkers, he falls back into his old, filthy habits.

Hmmmm, there's a message for me here somewhere. I honestly hadn't compared myself to Mark in this light before. I need to rid myself of my fat-promoting habits. I, too, need to keep myself as clean and made-up as possible each day, to give myself that little edge that helps keep me on my diet! Ha! Without even meaning to, I've described my own Daily

Checklist. I can get my whole life in order if I will merely follow my program.

Wednesday, January 25, 1989
228 pounds

I love the fact that I am into virgin fat, fat that I haven't lost and regained ten times in the last three years. I mean the solid, rock-bottom fat that has settled into ungiving, clinging, tenacious blobs all over my body. I am *never* going to have to lose these last forty-four pounds again.

It's fun to "think thin" again! It's too horrible when I'm eating out of control and gaining weight daily. At that terrifying point, I have no hope, so visualizing myself thin is generally depressing. But now, on my way down the scale, it's a wonderful prospect.

Saturday, January 28, 1989
229 pounds

Yesterday I baked and frosted a cake, even placing M&M's on top, without taking one little bite. Am I good, or what? Although I will admit that the night before, when I bought those M&M's, I was sorely tempted. In fact, I finally propelled myself from the kitchen because I knew I had to get away from the temptation.

The important thing is, I was able to mentally talk myself out of eating. I remained rational, though I was tempted to rip into that bag of M&M's. I had the sense and courage to get myself out! Like Joseph of old, when Potiphar's wife tried to seduce him, "and he left his garment in her hand, and fled, and got him out" of a compromising situation, I *ran* out of that kitchen.

Then yesterday, I geared myself up for the task of working with chocolate frosting and M&M's. I made myself talk to

Allen about the ordeal ahead of me. I needed to know he'd be checking on me. By fortifying myself, I made it through.

Allen keeps telling me I'm looking better. Oh, how I need his encouragement. But my situation is pathetic. Even when I lose fifty more pounds, I'll still be clinically obese and disgustingly fat—not exactly a pleasant thought. This is one long row to hoe! But believe me, when I'm done, I'm *never* going to let those stinkin' weeds grow again!

> *February 19, 1992. I am constantly learning from myself as I read my diary. I read about the difficulty I had in making that birthday cake, and I shake my head in disbelief. Why in the world did I ever make it in the first place? I am wiser now. I don't make anything that is hard for me to resist. Why should I? No one would ever expect an alcoholic to serve fancy alcoholic beverages to his guests. Why should I feel obligated to make fancy desserts for mine? No more. Yes, I am wiser: I refuse!*

Tuesday, January 31, 1989
229 pounds

Today has been sheer hell, starting with the first thing in the morning: weighing myself. Crud! Two hundred and twenty-nine pounds. I'm supposed to weigh 199 for Palm Springs. How can I lose thirty pounds in eight days? I am so frustrated. I don't know if I'll have the courage to go to Palm Springs.

Wednesday, February 1, 1989
229 pounds

I made it! I controlled myself today, even though I stupidly whipped up a batch of cookies. I was craving one of those cookies. Oh, who am I kidding? I was craving a dozen of those cookies, but instead of taking a nibble, I took control.

Tonight, someone remarked on my "fabulous skin"! I love compliments. But let's face it, at 229 pounds, I don't get too many about my looks! Allen tells me I have beautiful skin, and sometimes I laughingly reply, "It's a good thing, because skin is one thing I have *lots* of." Skin! I abhor this hangy fat roll. I guess I need to remember back to when I had several hangy fat rolls. It helps make the one roll that's left a little easier to bear. But boy, am I ready to let it go. I am ready to cut it off and send it to the moon.

I've lost forty-three pounds. And yet, I have to deal with this horrible reality: I look in the mirror and cannot dismiss this humongous human being staring back at me. I can't help wondering . . . is it actually possible for me to be thin again? Can my body ever recover?

Tuesday, February 21, 1989
232 pounds

I was desperate to weigh 199 by the time I went to Palm Springs. As each day passed, I became more and more frantic for success. I simply *could not* go to one of the most posh resort cities in America looking so fat.

At this point, the psyche of the fat person becomes fascinating. Okay. You have this intense struggle for weeks. Over and over you repeat to yourself, "Control your intake. Control your intake." Then, finally, you acknowledge that it is impossible—without liposuction—to lose your desired amount of weight before the deadline. So, do you determine to at least lose *something* before the big day? Do you earnestly vow to forge valiantly onward in your weight-reduction program? To lose those miserable extra pounds after all? Even if not in time for that special program, party, reunion, or whatever? *Suuuure* you do!

No, you quit your diet with a resounding, "I'm outta

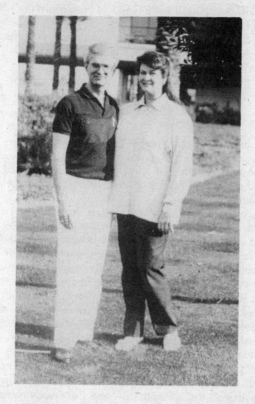

February 1989, 230 pounds. At Palm Springs—Allen as trim as
when we married, and me? At my goal of 199 . . . plus 31 pounds!
What a disappointment.

here!'' And you drive to the closest store, with your arms
open wide, ready to embrace the nearest candy, cookies,
pizza, cheese puffs, or German chocolate cake to your ample
bosom. You're not going to reach your goal, right? So why

try at all? And poor li'l you—you've been depriving yourself for so long. Go ahead and enjoy!

Here's one girl who refuses to justify any more binges. I refuse to get any deeper into debt with my own fat.

Tuesday, March 7, 1989
236 pounds

I am in an absolute "limbo" state of mind. I have been depressed, unorganized, unhappy. My mind seems to be full of cobwebs. Nothing is clear. I have accomplished zilch around the house. Yet my desire to change is overwhelming. My soul aches for it.

I have been devilishly sick the last three nights. I cannot believe a human being with an even vaguely working brain would do to herself what I have done. I went grocery shopping Saturday and bought five candy bars, exclusively for me. I ate them all within ten minutes of arriving home. I also bought a one-pound box of Whoppers. A one-pound box! I ate most of the Whoppers within moments of downing the candy bars.

Then I was struck by a generous (or could it be guilty?) impulse. I decided to share a few of the remaining Whoppers with Allen, Jenny, and Tiffany. I counted fifteen each into sandwich bags for them. The four of us were going to the school play in which Jeremy had the lead. Of course, I packed myself a sandwich bag of Whoppers, too. Only mine held more than all theirs combined—and I'd already eaten most of the box!

I am ashamed to admit that the only reason I shared even one Whopper was to keep my family from smelling chocolate on my breath. If they were eating some, too, I would blend in with the crowd. And who would know that I had more candy than anyone else? In the dark auditorium, no one could count. Even in a well-lit room, Whoppers are a terrific "sneaker" candy.

"What is a *sneaker* candy?" you ask. If you have to ask,

you are probably not fat. You can probably eat whatever you want, whenever you want, without worry of someone seeing fat ol' you eating again! That's why Whoppers are so handy for the fatty. You can sneak one plump Whopper through your lips with ease. No one notices!

When I arrived home from the play that night—oh, I am so embarrassed—I ate a whole box of Girl Scout cookies. I ate every last one of those chocolate-covered Caramel Delights! There were only fourteen cookies in the box, but they were overly rich, like candy bars.

I *knew* when I opened the box that I would eat each and every cookie. Even more important: *I knew when I opened the box that I would be getting disgustingly sick from it!* I *knew!* Yet I proceeded to open it. (Stop! *Stop!* You're taking that last step over the edge of the cliff. Don't open the box and you'll be okay!)

Brother, did I get sick! It started in the middle of the night. I tossed. I turned. I tried not to vomit. I almost "drank" Rolaids. I was so ashamed, so ashamed. And yet . . . I did it again—only forty-eight hours later.

Early yesterday afternoon, I bought (and quickly devoured) four candy bars. Then last night, when the children were in bed and Allen was working downstairs in his office, I ate another whole box of Girl Scout cookies—this time Thin Mints. There are twenty-one cookies in each Thin Mints box. I kept telling myself that eating *mint* cookies was kinda like eating Rolaids. Surely I wouldn't get sick from mint! Ha! My stomach was churning so violently last night, it could have made butter. My intense nausea kept me awake for hours.

I will *never* do that again. *Never!* I am thirty-six years old. I refuse to ever again gorge on goodies to the point of nausea. Here and now, I stop this downward descent that leads directly to misery and slavery. Talk about the gaping jaws of hell! I've been hanging over them long enough. This poor, frayed rope to which I am clinging cannot possibly hold one more ounce of me.

Wednesday, March 8, 1989
232 pounds

I was perfect today till Allen brought home some (sky darkens, thunder claps, lightning strikes) Winchell's doughnuts. I don't even *like* Winchell's doughnuts. They always leave a greasy coating in my mouth and another globule of greasy blubber on my middle, but I managed to down three. Then I opened another box of (won't I ever learn?) Girl Scout cookies. This time, I won't get sick. Relatively speaking, my total garbage count for today is not that high. But, boy, am I frustrated with myself! I wanted to lose another two pounds. (Is there a psychiatrist in the house?)

> *February 20, 1992. Rereading the above entry, I shook my head in disbelief. "Can you believe that, Allen? I did it again. I ate another box of Girl Scout cookies." He responded, "You wrote that you opened another box, but did you eat the whole thing?" I replied with a sneer on my face, "Was the box open? Think about it. I've never left a half-full box of Girl Scout cookies in the house in my whole life!"*

Thursday, March 9, 1989
230 pounds

My friend Jessica is a butterball, if ever there was one. She is very short and *very* round. She recently joined Weight Watchers and lost a few pounds. I am glad for her.

At a recent women's social at church, Jessica commented, "Guess what I had for dinner? Ab-so-lute-ly *nothing*!" No one responded to poor, little, starving-to-death Jessica's announcement of having eaten no dinner. So after a few minutes, she added, "I didn't eat any dinner because last week I gained a half-pound, and I know why." (Yes, Jessica, we *all* know why!) "It's those Girl Scout cookies." I had to laugh out loud because I, too, gorged on them. Probably half of the Girl Scout cookies sold are purchased by the fat moms of Girl Scouts! Clever of those Girl Scout cookie people.

I questioned Jessica about the number of cookies she'd eaten. "Around six." I almost choked on a snort!

I asked, "And that's the *only* thing you ate last week that wasn't on your diet?"

"Yes, that's all."

Then I became too honest without thinking about the consequences. "Oh, come on, Jessica. There's no way you'd gain half a pound from six little cookies—a total of only four hundred and eighty calories—if you were perfect on the rest of your diet."

"Oh, yes, I was!" (Very emphatically, maybe even a little huffily.)

At this point, I had sense enough to drop it. But please! What kind of diet would result in a half-pound weight gain from 480 extra calories? One must consume some 3,500 calories to gain one pound. Sorry, Jessica, "Methinks thou dost protest too much!"

I'm afraid Jessica was unable to be honest with herself. I don't think that she was deliberately lying. I believe she was using a common self-defense mechanism of fat people. It's the only way we foodaholics can survive sometimes. But here's one foodaholic who refuses to kid herself. That's why I make myself list everything I eat each day. It's not a pretty picture, but I make myself list it, even when I pig out.

Sunday, April 9, 1989
240 pounds

I am tired of this depression. But I can never be happy as an obese slob. I have to lose weight! Lose it and bury it and jump on the ground. Plant an oak tree over it, so its roots will go deep and keep that ugly, yellow, globby fat buried forever.

Okay. New day, new week, relatively new month, brand-new season. It's spring! Lovely time of year. New hope in the air. I will fill my lungs with it. (It's about time to fill *something* besides my stomach.)

I'm going to start a visual aid in my home. I'm going to start saving margarine boxes. I'm going to keep a stack of them where I can see them. Each pound I lose will be represented by one empty margarine box. My stack is going to grow like wildfire.

I am beginning to feel optimistic again through the magic of my pen. It writes hope for me. It spells out freedom. It inscribes dreams and goals, and soon, the reality of a thin me.

Monday, April 10, 1989
242 pounds

Years ago, one of my best friends, Marilynn Leavenworth, and I decided to start a "diet club." The club was a sincere attempt at doing something worthwhile and constructive about our weight. Marilynn did the inviting; I just couldn't. (What was I going to say? "Hi. I'm having a meeting for fat people, and, sister, you're at the top of my list!")

But Marilynn found it an easy task because she is refreshingly open and honest. She can also keep a confidence, so I could always trust her with my deep, dark secrets . . . like the secret of Rose's.

Okay, I admit it. We went to Rose's Restaurant a few times too many. They make these gargantuan pastries. I don't mean large, or even huge; I mean, they are gargantuan! Although most of their pastries are rather mediocre, we once had the good (or could it be horrible?) fortune to happen upon their Florentiners. Then their Napoleons. I would be willing to drown in a Florentiner or Napoleon and be thankful for the experience!

One is divinely chocolate, and the other is heavenly cream. My eyes are rolling even as I write. My mouth is watering this very moment. If you value your waistline, never, never order either one of them! Marilynn and I embraced them with all our hearts.

Once we drove to Rose's Take-Out Deli and ordered a Napoleon and a Florentiner . . . apiece! Remember, these are no small desserts. Yet I was standing at that counter worried that two huge, rich, calorie-packed desserts might not be enough to satisfy my intense craving of the moment. Afraid of starving to death, I ordered a fifth dessert to split between us. We then stopped at a corner store, bought a quart of milk to share, parked our car, and pigged out.

We both ate till we were sick to our stomachs. But heaven forbid we throw away one bite of those divine/diabolical concoctions. No, we ate every crumb! We licked our fingers. We picked every particle out of the sack and off the car seat. The only evidence we left of our dastardly deed was written all over our bodies.

We laugh about it today, but it was a disgusting display of gluttony. It was that kind of out-of-control eating that led us in desperation to start our famous diet club.

At our first meeting, nine hefty women showed up. We are talking major poundage here. Over one ton of beef (pork?) walked through my front door that night!

We had a plan. We were trying. Collectively, we lost forty-some pounds the first week. We were a roomful of desperate women. We laughed a lot, told on ourselves, and reported on our progress.

Marilynn still cracks up over one particular member's weekly report. This woman was the most honest, straight-arrow, truthful, trustworthy woman I knew—until it was her turn to give a progress report. She consistently announced either a few pounds lost or a break-even week. Yet Marilynn distinctly remembers the woman getting bigger and bigger, fatter and fatter. Poor thing. I know only too well the terror she felt. Sometimes it is impossible to admit a weight gain. We somehow talk ourselves into believing no one is noticing.

Like most diets, our club eventually fizzled out. But I give us credit for trying. And I do have some funny memories. The first night, moments before the initial meeting, Marilynn and I became panic-stricken. What? Us, diet? Before anyone came, we rushed to the store in a frenzy and bought some pastry. Back home, hiding in the kitchen, with *diet-club* women right in the next room, we stuffed it into our mouths. We laughed and kept telling each other: "This is it. No more sweets after tonight." We were laughing at ourselves and choking on the pastry. It was pathetic. It was certainly not funny. But laughter is not just the best medicine, sometimes it is the *only* medicine! We frantically wiped off any traces of our grievous sin before we marched into that roomful of fat ladies and tried to convert them to dieting. We both faked it well.

The thinner I get, the more I can laugh at that episode. It's hard to seriously laugh over fat antics while your chin is fluttering like a flag in a windstorm!

Tuesday, April 11, 1989
239 pounds

Today I was inspired to compose the words to my own diet song. This is not some mediocre ditty. Picture it being sung to the glorious tune of "The Impossible Dream." Bette Midler could put the correct feeling into it because she, too, has had to fight the disgusting battle. Of course, she's never had the extreme problem I have. But being in the limelight, she surely knows the agony of too many chocolates. Anyway, let's visualize Bette putting her heart and soul into this as only she can:

To lose the impossible pound,
To fight that disgusting last roll,

To spurn any pizza or cheesecake,
To run where no chocolate dare stroll.
To right the unrightable thigh,
Start today; it is never too late.
Don't stop, though you've had it with lettuce . . .
To lose the unlosable weight!
This is my dream, I want to be thin.
No matter how hopeless, I'll be there again!
To fight for my waist, it would be a delight!
To be willing to march into hell to have less cellulite!
And I know, if I'll only be true to this glorious goal,
That my heart will grow stronger for this . . .
    and quit paying the toll.
And the world will be better for this:
That one girl, fat and sick with self-hate,
Still strove with her last ounce of courage
To lose the unlosable weight!

(On some far-off day, I dream of singing this on Johnny
Carson's *Tonight Show*. Hey, I said it was a dream! Might
as well dream big!)

Wednesday, April 12, 1989
240 pounds

Tonight my head is nearly exploding with pain from an intense
toothache. Yikes! I'm going to call the dentist tomorrow and
see if I can make an emergency appointment. As I tell my
children, there are pros and cons to everything. And the pro
in this case? At least I don't feel like eating! We are talking
acute pain here.

Today I experienced "diet mania." I thought diet, I talked
diet—for crying out loud, I sang diet. The lyrics to the diet
song I wrote yesterday work famously. They pulled me
through today without a hitch. If I have to, I'll sing them in
the store while standing in front of the candy rack. I'll sing

them at the top of my lungs. After all, I can't very well stuff candy in my mouth while I'm singing. Finally, after sixteen years. I'm going be thin. Thin again.

Monday, May 1, 1989
241 pounds

Last night I watched an uplifting, motivating TV movie. It depicted the life of the founder of Alcoholics Anonymous. This man said a few things that truly inspired me, the most dramatic being the following declaration to his wife: "The most important thing in my life is staying sober." She asked, obviously hurt by the remark, "More important than me or our marriage?" He didn't answer yes, but quietly restated, "I *have* to stay sober."

I understand. It's true for me, too. The most important thing in my life right now is losing weight. I *have* to lose weight. Everything must take a backseat. As soon as I let other things keep me from taking care of me, *presto chango*, I'm off my diet.

Since I quit doing my program, I have become so depressed that I want to die again. Somehow, I must make it through this day. "One day at a time" was another important concept the founder of AA kept uppermost in his mind.

Thursday, May 4, 1989
236 pounds

I've written three diet songs to sing and use as inspiration. My main concern right now is my buddy. I need one. The wisest choice would be a thin person who has been fat before. The problem with having another fat person for a buddy is that if she doesn't stick to *her* diet, she usually gets mean and negative about *my* diet.

A negative buddy is incapable of providing the kind of

inspiration I need, like "Stick to it, Rose. Just today. You can make it. You can! Tomorrow morning, you will be so happy, so proud. Remember this: no matter what you eat today, good or bad, it will be over and done with by tonight. When you go to bed, it will be either with good food or with garbage in your body. The sweet tastes will be gone, a thing of the past. Don't make yourself sad tonight for what you eat today." Any person who has lost weight should be glad to help another weary traveler down the hard and sometimes hellish road. Hopefully, I can help others down that road someday.

Tuesday, May 16, 1989
236 pounds

What a struggle! It will never end. Like the alcoholic, I must make a conscious effort every day—for the rest of my life. An effort to think thin. An effort to work my program.

Last Thursday, I helped chaperon a field trip for Tiffany's school class. Didn't do my Daily Checklist first. Didn't think out lunch. Didn't commit to Allen to be good. It hit me like a ton of bricks, *Pow!* Eat, eat, eat! The second the children in Tiffany's class opened their lunches. I was surrounded by more Twinkies, chips, cookies, and treats than one sees in an hour of prime-time TV commercials! I wasn't prepared for it. I began to have a real, I-need-sweets-any-sweets attack. I could hardly wait to deliver those little children back to school, so I could race to the nearest neighborhood store and scarf to my heart's content. And I did.

I'm going to put a copy of my food list on the fridge each day. I need a reminder in the kitchen of what I get to eat for that day. I need to be sure I make my food list each morning. I should get my Jell-O made, my Alba in the freezer, my carrots and apples sliced. I need to be ready for any emergency! A baked chicken leg or two wouldn't be a bad idea, either.

Saturday, May 20, 1989
233 pounds

I've been sick for three days. When I'm in PJs all day, I tend to wander into the kitchen and eat anything that's not crawling, fuzzy, or fermented. I've tried to stay away from the kitchen altogether, but it's been hard.

I've been thinking some more about my rather pathetic childhood eating habits. For example, Mom and Dad would go to the Franz Bakery Thrift Store and buy volumes of bread, fruit pies, bear claws, and other pastries. The bread went swiftly into the freezer while the fruit pies, bear claws, and pastries went swiftly into our mouths. We ate them right out of the grocery bags. Before dinner. Before the bags of bread were unloaded. It used to upset Mom that we ate dessert first, but Dad was a voracious sweet eater, and since he started with dessert, so could we.

As a young girl, I was the recognized cookie maker of my family. I have always been a good cook, one of the major curses of my life. I don't know how many times I pulled out the biggest bowl we owned and doubled or tripled a cookie recipe. I knew exactly how many times I could multiply each recipe and still allow all the ingredients to fit into that bowl.

No matter how large a batch I made, there were never any leftover cookies! *Never!* Our cookie jar was purely for decoration. When I pulled the cookies out of the oven, my family often burned their fingers grabbing those irresistible, calorie-packed morsels off the hot cookie sheet. I can visualize the scene in my mind as if it were yesterday. I'd bend over to pull the cookie sheet out of the oven, and five or six people would crowd around me, each grabbing one or two cookies. Before I could turn from the oven to the kitchen counter, my cookie sheet was empty. I would reload it with more precious dough (which had been heavily dipped into by an assortment of fingers, mine included) and put another cookie sheet into the oven . . . only to experience the same crowd ten minutes later, licking their hot fingers. Often, that would happen to the whole double or triple batch of cookies.

That's where I first learned to down a cup of dough and two dozen cookies in one hour. I'd snitch the dough one quick glob at a time, and I'd eat my share of the cookies right out of the oven . . . or someone else would!

Tuesday, May 23, 1989
229 pounds

Tomorrow is my eighteenth wedding anniversary. That includes seventeen fat years! I am thankful that I am feeling some control in my life. The constant terror of being out of control makes me miserable. It is a continual source of amazement to me that I can turn from such depths of agony to try again. Sometimes the only thing that keeps me going, keeps me trying again, is the fact that I have a spark of the divine within. When I reach out to my Creator, I experience a never-ending hope. Without hope, life is meaningless.

I'm afraid life *had* become meaningless for two boys that went to school with my children. In the last two weeks, both boys, from two different schools, committed suicide. How my heart ached for their mothers, fathers, and families, but especially for their mothers. What agony those mothers must have experienced. I wept hot, sorry tears for them both, and for the poor, little, lost lives.

Jeremy knew one of the boys. He was in two of Jeremy's high-school classes. This boy hadn't been especially popular; he was a little quiet, a little unsure of himself. His hair was often slightly greasy and was not cut in the latest style. His shirts were a little too small, his pants a little too short.

I keep torturing myself with the thought that maybe if one person had said hi to him that day; if one student had asked, "Hey, can I sit with you for lunch?"; if one teacher had complimented, "John, you did much better on your last assignment," maybe . . . maybe he wouldn't have felt compelled to end his sad, young life. Maybe he needed only one tiny reason to want to live. Maybe he required just one ray of hope, one hand of friendship to feel that at least today was better than yesterday.

I guess those two boys had a sort of hope . . . a hope for a better existence, perhaps. A hope for some rest or peace or love or acceptance. Please, God, help them find it. Take them to your forgiving heart and help them find some comfort and love in the eternities. And please . . . give solace to their poor, grieving mothers.

I pray that someday I will be able to make a difference in someone's life, that I can give someone hope for success on this earth. I want to help people reach their potential by ridding themselves of life-sucking fat. And, if I ever get rich, I want to establish some kind of "anti-geek" center offering classes where kids can learn social survival skills: how to dress, how to walk, how to keep as clean and good-looking as possible—whether rich or poor, fat or thin.

Friday, May 26, 1989
224 pounds

Yesterday I talked with Allen about how important it is for me to have a buddy. I need someone to report to. I need someone to buoy me up. I need someone to exult with. He made grandiose promises of helping me. He filled me with so much hope for the future, I thought I would burst.

Now, when you float around in that big of a bubble, believe me, the pop hurts! Our agreement was perfectly clear. Be ready for bed by 10:30—in our pajamas, with teeth brushed and flossed. But could he do it for one night? Could he help his own wife, who was deathly sick with a disease as life-threatening as cancer? Seventeen years sick? Heavens, no.

The lesson to learn here is this: I will never again count on him to give me the support I need. Although I've felt that way before, yesterday I foolishly believed him. Somehow, his sweet talk sucked me in again. Oh, it's so hard. Who can I turn to? There is no one, yet I drastically need someone. It would be nice to have one real friend.

Above and beyond this hurt, I am determined to do well today. I will show this whole world that I am a genuine person, not just a roly-poly piece of Play-Doh! I love my songs. I sing them all day long. I want to write more. I need to record them so I can play them constantly. They lift me up and give me hope and support. Maybe I can be my own buddy.

Tuesday, May 30, 1989
226 pounds

Yesterday I ate entirely too much at an all-you-can-eat restaurant. I begin with beautiful goals. I enter that buffet line totally committed to my diet, determined that this time I will analyze and be superbly selective about every ounce that I put on my plate. Then, somehow, the food mysteriously appears on my tray. Why, *I* certainly don't mound up all that bulk to voluntarily take into my own body. And heaven forbid I should waste it! So what do I do? I *waist* it. After all, I'm entitled to as much as I want. I'm going to get my $5.39 worth, if it kills me!

On a positive note, I had only two small cinnamon rolls for dessert. I quit before I was so full I became nauseated. For me, that's an accomplishment. But I will not (Do you hear me, world? *Will not!*) go there again till I weigh 175 or less.

How can anyone be so totally neglectful as Allen is of me? I told him ahead of time I didn't want to go to that restaurant. But his parents had offered to treat us to an all-you-can-eat buffet, and he found it difficult to suggest a different place.

All one has to do is take a good look around that restaurant and observe the typical clientele. We are talking major hulks here. At least half the people are dangerously obese. Some of them make me feel dainty. It is definitely not a pretty picture. I find myself humiliated whenever I go there. I am forced to come face to face with those huge people and their huge plates of food. I abhor being one of them, but our fat ties us together as surely as having the same grandpa would.

In spite of my disgust, I manage to wolf down a huge plateful. I have my children go back for my seconds and thirds and often fourths. I brainwash myself into believing "It's okay, it's only chicken. Only shrimp. Only my first dessert. Only the second time I've eaten out this month." Of course, the chicken and shrimp are breaded and deep-fried. Get real, Rose. Thank goodness I had the courage to tell Allen (even as I write) to not take me there again till I can see an honest 175 pounds on my scale.

That was Monday. After all that gorging and self-disgust, how did I do today? I devoured eight Otis Spunkmeyer chocolate chip cookies, okay? Eight! How I hate that man. That blackguard. That purveyor of cruelty. I almost drool thinking about Otis Spunkmeyer chocolate chip cookies. I dream of them. They are divine. I hate Otis Spunkmeyer!

Wednesday, May 31, 1989, 9:30 A.M.
224 pounds

I am just sick. Elizabeth Taylor is fat again. It scares me to death. It is depressing. I cannot imagine anyone so beautiful, so glamorous, so rich, being so fat. But worse, she had fought the good fight and won! She was down to a size five, for crying out loud. My upper *arm* is as big as a size-five waist! Then, battle by battle, pound by pound, she fell to the enemy. It is disappointing. I cried the first time I saw her fat again. To think that she's in the limelight and still couldn't cut it. For heaven's sake, what hope is there for the rest of us fatties? Those who don't have a public to appear before?

When I saw her on *Oprah* awhile back, she was gorgeous and glamorous and thin. I was eating my heart out during the whole interview over a woman twenty years older than I am. At one point, Oprah asked her what finally made her click into gear and lose all the weight. Elizabeth Taylor replied, "I stopped in my dressing room and stood in front of a mirror. And it was there hanging out. I had no clothes on, and I looked at it all and said, 'That's not pretty . . . *now* is the time.'"

Oprah: "That's interesting, because you'd seen it before. You'd seen yourself before."

Elizabeth: "Yeah, but I'd managed to fleet. You know, just sort of flit and just catch a fleeting glance of somebody moving. . . . That blob was . . . was . . . that blob wasn't me."

So she lost every ugly fat cell on her body. Oh, Elizabeth, you were my inspiration. Now what will I do? I keep telling myself, "She can afford fresh crab legs in her fridge! For crying out loud, she can afford a food guard." She could hire someone to watch over her twenty-four hours a day and keep her out of the kitchen. Why doesn't she do it? Here I am, trying to squeeze $1.13 out of my budget for a frozen dinner (260 calories), and she wears diamonds that could buy me a lifetime supply. I don't get it. But I know she can do it again!

Two Sundays ago, I saw an old acquaintance. She must have lost eighty pounds since the last time I saw her. She was massive before, so she still needs to lose another forty pounds. Still overweight, she insisted on pulling a too-typical fat-person trick: she wore a gathered skirt and a bulky blouse . . . tucked in! I will *not* tuck in a blouse till I have a flat stomach. I will not! Why proclaim to the world that your stomach pouches out like the muscles on Popeye's arms?

January 29, 1991. I saw that same old acquaintance again last Sunday. The poor woman found every last pound she had lost! And it's been only a year and a half. A year and a half! What a bummer. It is scary for me. This is a lifelong experience, this dieting business. I must never forget that.

Same day, 2:16 P.M.

I am so hyped up right now—I'm floating on cloud ten! By comparison, this high is even higher than my last low was low. When I walked into Debbie's backyard today, all three of my sisters—Barbara, Debbie, and Rebecca—were there. Rebecca turned around and said, "Hey! Have you just lost a ton of weight or something?" Barb said, "You do look a lot better." Oh yes, yes, yessss! I wanted someone to notice. It's so stupid. It's as if until someone comments on your weight loss, you haven't really lost weight. It sounded great, like soda pop pouring over ice on a hot day.

Thursday, June 1, 1989
220 pounds

Another new month. How can life fly by like this? But everything seems better when I'm losing weight. I squeezed out another four pounds on the scale this morning. Sometimes I feel so silly standing there, shifting my weight, trying to maneuver the numbers down, but I can't help myself. The fatty learns exactly where and how to stand on the scale in order to find the lowest reading. Isn't that ridiculous? But we all do it.

Hey! I've lost fifty-two pounds. The most I've ever lost before on one sustained diet was sixty-five pounds. Of course, that time I didn't begin my dieting at 272 pounds. I started at 215 and ended at 150. One hundred and fifty. Yup! I looked pur-ty good! Will I ever be there again? Yes! And sometime during the year 1989!

Friday, June 2, 1989
224 pounds

I am feeling heavily depressed; I don't think even four Otis Spunkmeyer cookies could lift my spirits today. But I'm about ready to give old Otis a try. My poor mother tried for years to lift some of the bleakness out of her life through goodies. She frequently sent one of us children on excursions to our little neighborhood store, with her famous "*You know what I want.*" It was her secret message that she was craving a "U-No" candy bar. Mom would call one of us in and say she needed a loaf of bread or a gallon of milk or a box of baking soda, and "*you know* what I want." She would raise her eyebrows in a certain, meaningful way and establish intense eye contact as she verbally underscored "you know." She could send that secret code around Dad or the little kids, and they wouldn't understand.

As I reviewed my diary and came face-to-face with my own sick behavior, I had a sudden realization. Mother often *pretended* to need items at the store in order for one of us children to get her a "*you know* what"! And I have done the same type of clever finagling with my own children. It makes me sad and ashamed.

I must be the one who finally disposes of this ugly legacy. Today I vow to never again ask my children to buy anything sweet for me. At least it's a beginning.

Friday, June 16, 1989
216 pounds

I "exposed" a little part of myself to my mother-in-law last Monday night. I shared a small portion of my diet program, including my diary. I even showed her (oh, pity the woman) some of my *fat* pictures. Ha! The pictures aren't so fat, but I sure am. Picture this: a 248-pound woman—in a swimsuit!

Yuck, gag, and all the other words I can think of for regurgitating. This is not a pretty picture!

It's scary to think of "exposing" myself to another person. Not just showing my pictures, but totally exposing my heart and soul, my ideas and dreams. It's terrifying. What happens if I show someone these gross pictures of me and then I get as fat again? They'll know what I look like! What a nightmare! But I won't get fat again! I am on my program for life.

Two days ago, I was especially frustrated that I am fat! I walked into Mervyn's to buy a dress for Jenny's eighth-grade graduation. We found several darling dresses for her to try on, selected her favorite, and headed innocently to pay for it when, *whammo*, we were subjected to pornography at the cash register. There on display were packages of intimate women's underwear featuring an eight-by-ten-inch cover picture of a beautiful, *well-built*, nearly naked young woman in a sexy pose.

We had walked into Mervyn's family clothing store, for crying out loud. We were not prepared to have pictures of a naked woman thrust at us as we paid for our purchases.

If I were thin, I would feel much more like raising hell over such issues, but because I'm fat, I'm afraid everyone will think I'm just jealous. I did express my anger to the lady at the cash register. She didn't like the picture either, but there was "nothing she could do about it." Phooey! We can all do a lot more than we think. Well, although I didn't have the nerve (it's hidden by too much fat) to go to customer service and give them a piece of my mind, at least I mailed in an official complaint. But, boy-oh-boy, I can hardly wait for "my day in court"—the day I will feel good enough about me that I can stand up for modesty without being perceived as someone merely frustrated with her own fat.

January 29, 1991. I need to note here that I did receive a letter from Mervyn's in response to my complaint. They were concerned and apologized. They moved the display to the back of the store and

*said they would talk to the company that produced
the product to see about changing the picture.*

On the *Sally Jessy Raphael Show*, I saw a man who has
lost 694 pounds. With only twenty more to reach his goal,
he's done it in seventeen months. Wow!

On Sally's show, the question was asked many times in
many ways, "What can a loved one do to help?" Of course,
there's the proverbial "Don't *nag*." Followed by "There is
nothing you can do until the fatty decides to do something
him/herself." That is a blatant I-don't-take-the-time-
to-get-involved lie.

There *are* things people can do to help a fat spouse, friend,
or relative. Most fat people are honest enough to admit they
would like to lose weight. Talk about it with them. Tell them
you love them and want them around for a long time. Go out
of your way to read and discuss problems of the obese with
them and the advantages of being thin. Ask your fat loved
ones what you can do to help. Discuss their particular food
temptations and make a noble effort to keep those foods out
of the house.

Don't bring treats home for the "thin" family members.
Every time you do, the fatty instantly begins to plan and
scheme to sneak some of those treats the second your back
is turned. Just seeing snacks on the counter starts the saliva
running for a fatty. It starts a train of thoughts about food
that gains momentum with each passing minute. Pretty soon
that train of thoughts is careening down a mountain of scrumptious mental images until it crashes at the bottom in one huge
pig-out orgy!

Don't offer *any* food to someone who is obese. Believe
me, fat people don't need to be reminded to eat. Sometimes
your making the offer is all the fat person needs for an excuse
to inhale calories. When you go to a function of any kind,
discuss with your fat spouse or loved one exactly what she
plans to eat while away from home. Help her commit ahead
of time. She's worth the few minutes it takes. Don't go to

any fast-food restaurants because you're in a hurry. Insist on going somewhere that serves healthy, low-calorie meals. Remind her to bring along lo-calorie dressing, butter substitute, and diet pop.

Let her know you're thinking of her. Be aware of her eating fits. I pork out at night. If Allen had only said a few words to me last night before he went to his office to work: "Now, honey, I know this is a hard time of day for you. Please try to be strong. If you get the eating crazies, call me and talk first, and I'll try to talk you out of it. Is there anything more you plan to eat tonight?" Those words would have saved me over 1,000 calories yesterday. It's not Allen's fault that I overate, but he *could have helped* me control myself.

I don't expect thin people to fully comprehend the plight of a fat person, but when a fatty says she is going to try another diet, don't pooh-pooh the poor soul. Support her. Find out details of the diet and help by suggesting meals that will work. Help the fatty exercise. Exercise with her.

One last thought: Don't help for one or two days and then quit. Your lack of caring enough to follow through will signal a reason for an eating binge that rolls forth like a snowball down a steep hill. It usually takes years to get fat. It follows that it will probably take years to undo the damage, and then a whole lifetime to keep it under control.

Saturday, June 17, 1989
218 pounds

I am angry, hurt, and frustrated. Surely anyone who has lived with me for eighteen years should know better than to do what Allen did to me tonight.

Dinner hour was over in our happy little home. I had settled into my bedroom for the evening. Suddenly, little Tyler cried out those words that bring fear into the heart of any earnest dieter, "Mommy, I'm hungry." Oh, those dirty, diet-destroying words. I had been good today, and I didn't want to spoil a whole day's worth of earnest dieting. Could I possibly have the strength to fix him food without opening my mouth for one cookie crumb? Sure, I could always—no! I didn't have the strength. But did I have the courage to tell Allen I didn't have the strength?

"Allen!" I blurted it out as fast as my tongue could trip over the words. "Allen, Tyler wants something to eat, and I'm afraid to go into the kitchen because I'm afraid *I'll* eat." Phew! I said it. It was out!

Unbelievably, Allen didn't jump at the chance to fix Tyler some food, and, just maybe, save my diet. Jump, schmump! He didn't leap or walk or move one foot toward the kitchen. If I said he didn't lift his eyes from the newspaper, you might think that I was exaggerating. But he didn't, he didn't, didn't, didn't, didn't! And I had my excuse! Right then and there, I knew I was in for a real pig-out. I almost started tingling with anticipation. "Oh, never mind, Allen. I'll go fix him something. I'm kinda hungry, anyway."

Oh, you fool, Allen. All I needed was a little help. Some tiny acknowledgment of how strong I was trying to be. You're some support, Allen! Please help me! Why won't you help me? It seems impossible to succeed on my own.

Monday, June 19, 1989
213 pounds

Men! They are so dumb sometimes. At least where women and children are concerned . . . and other men and maybe animals and . . .

I'm feeling pretty good. I'm down three more pounds, for a total of fifty-nine. I wore a new blouse today. I even *feel* younger (in spite of my birthday yesterday, when I turned thirty-seven—boo!).

Today, my three sisters and I met at Debbie's house to celebrate my birthday belatedly. They commented on how good I was looking, that my new blouse was the perfect color for me. When I came home, I floated down to Allen's office, feeling quite cute and almost petite. Feeling on top of the world and full of hope. I practically sang out to Allen, "You can tell me how cute I am." With a smile on his face, the big dope said, "You do look cute. You look like a cute, little expectant mama!" One stupid, thoughtless sentence, and my hope vanished like gangbusters, my "cuteness" went up in smoke. I felt more like an elephant than anything near petite. My beautiful, new blouse that I "looked so good in" became a hateful, hideous old rag which I wanted to rip to shreds and dump on Allen's desk.

Writing about it makes me feel better, but I'll always hate this blouse I'm wearing, just the same.

Saturday, June 24, 1989
210 pounds

Last week was shot because I let a dumb dog's barking mess up my schedule for doing my checklist. So the neighbor's dog woke me up every day at 4:00 A.M. So I should have gotten up and exercised. Started early. Taken a shower. Made myself ready for the day. (And then, possibly, I should have gone out to buy a pellet gun for that stupid dog!)

About a week ago, I was grocery shopping. I am starting to feel thinner. My clothes fit more loosely, and my face is prettier, so I stand a little taller and smile a lot more. Well, there I was, smiling away while shopping, when suddenly I felt like I was living a line from my own poem. The line that goes:

I want to wear clothes and hats that would make
A handsome young man do a double take.

Okay. So the man wasn't exactly handsome. So the man wasn't exactly young. But he was a man, and he did an exceptional double take. In fact, he jerked his head back in my direction so hard, I was afraid he'd suffered whiplash. (How's that for laying it on thick?)

Anyway, it made me feel good. Silly, isn't it? (I guess every woman loves a compliment and never outgrows the craving for one.) After a second, I figured the whiplash guy must have thought I was someone he knew because—let's get rational here—I'm teeter-tottering at 210 pounds. By no stretch of the imagination can 210 pounds be whistle bait! But, when it happened again the *next* day, I thought maybe I was actually starting to look better. I was driving along, pulled up to a stoplight, and noticed the driver on my right glance at me and then whip his head back in my direction for a real, true double take. Incidentally, this man *was* young and handsome. Of course, I'm not completely loony. I'm aware that he could see only the best part of me, from my neck up. But, hey, a double take is a double take.

Last night I joined the ranks of the living again: I indulged myself in a little swimming at Dahl Park, on the Clackamas River. Let me tell you, no double takes there. Ouch! Going to the river meant I had to face the reality of . . . swimsuits. Swimsuit! That horrid S-word.

At my all-time highest weight, when I made the Incredible Hulk look sickly and malnourished, I was considerate of mankind and stayed away from swimming pools with the same dedication I gave to seeking out chocolate. It was an exciting moment when, having lost enough poundage to feel that my limbs were recognizable as human, I allowed myself the luxury of swimming. But I had the decency to wear shorts and a blouse. I spared mankind the full display of the disastrous consequences of my insatiable appetite.

If you are brave enough, I will now take you on a walk down misery lane. It begins in the swimming-pool dressing room. For the real fatty, squeezing into a swimsuit is a feat by itself. We are talking stuffed sausage here. It is humorous how one must pull, stretch, strain, tuck in fat, lift up rolls, and otherwise distort oneself to squeeze into one cubic foot of material.

Once one has suffered the personal degradation of trying

to get into a suit, one must now brave the gates of hell while stepping out of the dressing room and into public view. How one tries to walk tall. How one tries to hold in whatever part of her body over which she has any muscle control. How one strains her eyes to find at least one person a little fatter, a little more rippled than she.

And have you ever noticed how fat people are able to get used to the water so quickly? They never stand coyly on the pool steps, dipping in one red-lacquered toenail. They don't sit demurely on the side of the pool, one leg pulled up sexily beneath them, gently playing pat-a-cake with the water with their free foot. And they don't saunter through the shallow end, cockily turning their head from side to side to see who is noticing the latest swim fashion they are modeling.

No, we fat mamas barge into that water like a battleship plows through the high seas. We see no one. Our eyes are firmly fixed on the deep blue water before us, the deep blue refuge, where we can sink mercifully below the surface and feel some relief from the ugly stares of others and from our own, hideous bulges. For beneath the water, it's almost true that "all men are created equal." At least our fat doesn't feel as heavy and flabby while under water.

Once in the pool, we human buoys stay in till quitting time. It doesn't matter if we're hungry, thirsty, or turning into prunes. We stay in that pool till we've had our fill. Then, oh-so-carefully, we creep back to the shallow end. We pretend we're playing with our little ones as we use our hands to crawl along like waterdogs in the two-foot water. At the last possible second, we get up out of the water, trying frantically to pull the clinging suit away from our rolls and ripples without appearing too obviously distraught. We feel the whole world is staring at us through a magnifying glass. We have learned exactly how fast we can move without bouncing and jiggling too much. Oh, the long, drawn-out moments till we reach our towel and can breathe a sigh of relief.

Now, you will notice that we so cleverly brought along a beach towel. No little bathroom towel for us. Those extra-long, extra-wide beach towels are capable of covering a *bazil-*

lion candy bars and cookies. And, as when wearing a coat, we fool ourselves into thinking no one will notice how big we are once we're covered. And that, I guess, just about covers fat people and swimming.

Monday, June 26, 1989
213 pounds

It's been a good day. I felt Allen's support toward my diet for the first time in ages. This morning, he said he would skip work today and help me get organized, and then he actually *did* it. I feel high and hopeful. I can do it. I *will* be thin again.

Monday, July 10, 1989
219 pounds

When am I ever going to grow up and accept total responsibility for me? Allen can help, but if he doesn't call me for our meeting by 10:15 P.M., then I can call him. I *will* call him. I have been unbelievably stupid! Every night I go through the same dumb routine: I wait around, seeing if he'll come up for our meeting. Like a cat watching a mouse. Will he come? Ten-twenty—he should already be upstairs getting into his PJs. (*Suuuure* I can count on him this time.) Ten-twenty-three—he should be brushing his teeth. (But he doesn't love me or care about me. He's still in his office downstairs.) Ten-twenty-five—he hasn't even come out of his door. (It's all his fault I'm fat. No wonder I eat M&M's, no wonder I gorge on goodies! He can't give me twenty minutes a day!) Ten-twenty-eight—he should be flossing this minute. And now, ten-thirty—he did it again! No sign of him. My big support! My buddy! He failed me again. Soon he'll come hurrying up the stairs with some feeble line. "Was it ten-thirty we were supposed to meet?" or "What, you expected me to be ready for bed before our meeting?'' Or how about this doozie? ''But I didn't think you'd be ready yet, because I heard talking upstairs.''

Oh, please! Spare me the excuses. I've heard them all a thousand times. If I'd been a business meeting or church appointment, you would have been there with bells on. But I'm only me, your wife, the mother of your children, a day-care provider, a nothing, a zip, a zero. I don't blame you for not caring. Really, I don't. I don't think I'm worth the trouble either. So, I hereby pledge to myself that I will *never* blame Allen again for not keeping our appointments.

New strategy: *I* remind Allen each night by 10:15. *I* get myself ready for bed by 10:30. *I* have my workbook ready to go over with him. If *I* am ever to succeed, *I* must take charge of the situation. Sitting back and waiting for Allen to somehow organize my room, my schedule, my life, my mind is not just stupid, it's impossible. Only *I* know what's in my mind, and while Allen can support and help me, he is only an innocent bystander.

Thursday, August 10, 1989
236 pounds

I am so frustrated with myself, so tired of failure. Wise and learned men can speak all they want of ''not failing until you give up,'' but the reality of me, right now, this minute, weighing 236, is Failure with a capital *F*.

Some days I feel like giving up. It would be much simpler to adopt the philosophy, ''Eat, drink, and be merry, for tomorrow we die.'' But I can't. If I keep eating like this, tomorrow I really might die, and who could lift me into a coffin? Oh, horror of horrors!

There is yet a little spark of hope in me. An ounce of faith, a pinpoint of light. Yet the spark is becoming dim, the ounce dissolving fast, and the pinpoint closing up. I am so frightened! I want to be thin. It consumes my soul. Yet daily, hourly, I harbor evil, wicked thoughts of sweets and pastries and ice cream. Why can't I be normal? Why can't food be merely a source of nourishment for me? Why do I have to *live and breathe* for it? There has to be some synapse in my brain that is not "synapsing" properly. I want to quit thinking of food.

Today I read a magazine article entitled "Sage's Song" about an unusually beautiful little girl who was burned and disfigured into something barely recognizable as human. The pictures of little Sage were brutally honest. I wept as I read about her horrible accident. I ached to caress her little body. I longed to comfort her parents over the loss of the little Sage they had known.

Then I thought about me. What about me? A disfigurement of my *own* making! I knew this poor little five-year-old would surely give up candy bars to have her fingers or nose or ears back. Oh, little baby "monster," what food wouldn't you give up to be your former self again, to run and play as in days of old? I wish my acute sorrow could somehow help you, Sage. Your story has deeply touched my life. I, too, am grotesquely misshapen. Surrounded, not by scarred flesh, but by yellow, greasy globules of hanging, saggy flesh.

I can correct my deformity. Sage cannot. Thank you, Sage, for helping me to see clearly again. Someday, I will shake your dear little stump of a hand and bless your name. I am so ashamed of what I have voluntarily done to my once beautiful body.

Wednesday, October 18, 1989
245 pounds

Life has little meaning or hope. Television and books are my only escape from nothingness. This morning, as I wandered aimlessly around my house, wondering what to do, I couldn't help finding a little amusement in my ironic situation. Me, wondering what to do? Oh, please. Talk about having eyes but not seeing! My whole house is a disaster area. I won't try to describe the various messes in every room, yet I am wandering aimlessly around, wondering what to do. I strongly suspect that this type of behavior is a manifestation of depression. (Oh, depression! I *hate* that word! Just hearing that blasted word makes me depressed!)

I am tired of being frightened. I think I'm frightened of losing myself. (Not losing weight, mind you, but losing myself!) Some of me is dying each day. Pretty soon, all that will be left is a hollow shell. I want Rosemary back. I think maybe I am going crazy.

I have much to be thankful for, but that doesn't make it any easier. I feel all the more a worthless creep, because I have no right to be so depressed.

Where is all this taking me? To my Daily Checklist. I can touch it and write on it. It's not some ethereal idea. I can start at the top of my list and know what to do. I don't have to wander and wonder anymore. It is my last hope. Not to lose weight, as much as to find me. I haven't washed my hair for four days, or showered for three. Depression does that to me. One surefire way to fight the big "D" is to keep as clean and pretty as possible, so I'm off to the shower.

Wednesday, October 25, 1989
246 pounds

At ages thirteen and fourteen, Debbie and I had a memorable chocolate experience together. My family was attending a big church conference. There were hundreds of people in the building. Being a typical teenager, I was bored to death. Debbie and I had pulled that famous, you-leave-first-then-I'll-follow-in-a-few-minutes trick. When I walked into the ladies' room, there was Debbie, arguing with a couple of pretty tough-looking girls. Debbie was always one to be a little feisty.

Rosemary to the rescue: "What's going on here?"

First tough-looking girl: "What's it to you?"

Rosemary, rather firmly: "She's my little sister."

Second tough-looking girl: "Well, your little sister stole a candy bar out of my purse that I left in this bathroom."

Rosemary, sounding self-assured: "This is not a private bathroom. A lot of people have used this room today."

Second girl: "Yeah, well, we were only gone for a few minutes, and when we came back, your sister was alone in here. And I can smell chocolate on her breath."

Rosemary, condescendingly: "Of course you can smell chocolate. What do you think, that you were the only people in this whole crowd who thought to bring something to munch on today? I brought several packages of M&M's myself! Look, I know my sister. If she says she didn't eat your dumb candy bar, she didn't eat your dumb candy bar!" (I can be pretty feisty, myself.) I knew they couldn't prove anything. I took a deep breath, stood as tall as possible, stared them straight in the eyes, and stood my ground. They mumbled a few more words under their breath and left the rest room.

I spun around, squinted my eyes at Debbie, and hissed out, "Did you eat that candy bar?" (You bet I knew my sister! And I was pretty sure I knew where that missing candy bar was.)

All the feistiness left Debbie like a balloon with a fast leak. She suddenly looked smaller and deflated, almost whispering, "Yes, I ate it."

"Oh, you idiot! What in the world did you think was going to happen?"

Debbie, quickly regaining her composure and her snappy tongue: "I didn't think anyone would be coming back so soon for the purse, okay? I was only looking through the purse to see what the owner carried. I wouldn't have taken any money or anything. But when I saw that chocolate candy bar, it . . . jumped out at me and . . . and . . . I ate it. It wasn't my fault. They're the ones who left the dumb purse in here in the first place! Thanks for sticking up for me, Rose. Hey, could I have some of those M&M's?"

"Ya nuthead, Debbie, I don't have any M&M's! I made that up!"

"Wow! I believed you. You're good!"

As I look back on the experience, it's rather shameful. Oh, I can make it sound kind of funny, but the bottom line is, Debbie stole a candy bar, and I covered it up . . . at a church conference, no less! I never thought of it as an incredibly obvious symptom of an eating disorder. I knew at the time that her urge to eat that chocolate was nearly impossible to control. And now, some twenty-three years later, we are both still struggling with that same, terrible craving.

Monday, October 30, 1989
247 pounds

I like to visualize that dramatic scene in *Gone With the Wind* where Scarlett O'Hara holds her fist to the heavens and vehemently declares, "As God is my witness, I will never go hungry again!" At that moment, she felt an unquenchable determination coursing through her veins. I feel a similar force in my life this day. I have been beaten down at every turn; I am sick to death of the struggle. I have the solution, and so I, Rosemary Green, vehemently declare, "As God is my witness, I will fill in every square on my checklist today!"

Saturday, November 4, 1989
248 pounds

I have lived a gray, miserable, depressed week. I have felt "sickish" all day, every day. I haven't had the flu. I've had "yuck-I-ate-too-much-itis"! Don't ask me how I can do it to myself. There *is* no explanation. But this instant, every fat cell in my body is screaming out to be released.

I'm getting dizzy spells again. My back is constantly aching. My knees creak like crazy. This is hell.

Thursday, November 30, 1989
255 pounds

Today I had to dig my Daily Checklist out from a two-foot-high stack of papers on my desk. No wonder I've climbed back up to 255 pounds, more than I've weighed for a couple of years.

It is hard for me to comprehend being this fat. It is impossible for me to understand how it all came about. In searching for someone or something to hold accountable for the disgusting state of my body, I can't think of a better place to point the ugly finger of blame than at my marriage. When first married, I expected my husband to come home at 5:15 every day, just as I had seen my father do for eighteen years. But I didn't marry a truck driver, I married a corporate vice president. Corporate vice presidents don't come home at 5:15 every day. In fact, I can honestly say they never come home at 5:15.

After only a few months of marriage, my husband accepted a volunteer position in our church. It was a very time-consuming job, involving serious responsibility. He was also the steady drummer for two singing groups and one dance band, often performing twice a week. Night after night, week after week, month after month—yes, even year after year—he would rush in the front door, wolf down his dinner, and be out the door again in less than half an hour.

Many nights, I wept in my loneliness. Many more nights, I fell back on my childhood habits and chose to invite in questionable company. I had a full-fledged, illicit affair going with . . . chocolate and pastries and ice cream. I combined enough high-voltage calories with mushy love stories (either from books or TV) to cry and eat my way up to 300 pounds. My heart still goes out to that disillusioned, unfulfilled young woman who was me.

These heartrending memories are tragic for me, but the greatest tragedy of all is when we can't learn something from the miserable experiences of life. I have learned two important truths from this particular part of my past. First, the best children in the world can't take the place of a husband. Second, one cannot fill one's needs by filling one's mouth!

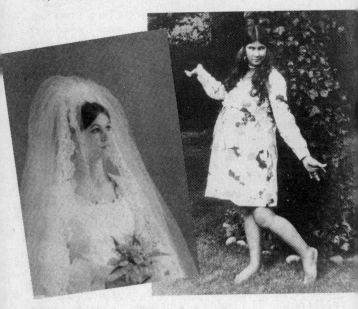

May 1971, 142 pounds, and September 1972, 210 pounds. And so it all began. On my wedding day, I had no idea I would look like this in sixteen short months! I ate to fill a void . . . and I created a mountain!

Friday, December 29, 1989
248 pounds

It's easy to look at other people and think, Why? Why doesn't that man brush his teeth? Why doesn't that woman wash or even comb her hair? Why doesn't that heavy teenage girl wear clothes that suit her plump figure? Why doesn't that family clean their house, or at least one room? Why don't those people remove the junk from their front yard? Why, why, why?

The truth of the matter is, I'm the biggest *why* of all. Why don't I quit making my own life miserable? Christmas Eve, I ate like a maniac, and Christmas day, I devoured a portion of every yummy morsel that tap-danced through my front door. (And since our Lind family gathering was at my house, my front door saw tons of yummy morsels!) I had more chocolate-coated, chocolate-filled, chocolate-flavored delights than I should have had in a whole month, knowing with every bite that I would get sick that night! Then I topped off that unsettling assortment with cookies, pastries, cakes, candied nuts, punch, a variety of cold cuts, chips, and dips. It was one continual eating fest!

Christmas night, I was so sick I wanted to die. I tossed and turned and thought I was going to vomit. So the next morning I swore to myself, "Not one sweet thing today." I swore it. I didn't say "diet"; but I swore to eat no garbage desserts. I didn't have the oomph, the commitment, the gumption to say "diet." I couldn't diet, but somehow I had to control my intake for the sake of sleep. I couldn't go through another miserable night. I made it for a whole half hour. Then my willpower deteriorated from "no sweets" to "no candy." There were plenty of noncandy sweets around. This is megadistressing to have to record. I hurriedly put down a half dozen cookies. I made it all the way to noon without any strictly defined candy, at which time I proceeded to "nibble" on fudge, peanut brittle, and anything else my nose upturned in its search for sweets. However, the total quantity I consumed was less than the day before, and I didn't feel as though I were going to vomit that night. But I still felt wretched. What a disgusting thing to have to write about myself.

Today, I decided to try earnestly one more time! Among other reasons, I have only one dress, one pair of pants, and one blouse that fit me. Eighteen measly pounds, and my wardrobe doubles or triples. Thirty-five pounds, and my wardrobe multiplies by six or eight times. I can't afford new clothes. So lose eighteen pounds, I must!

At this moment I feel strong. It seems so simple. So obvious. In a few short weeks, I could be a new person, mentally and physically. I could have a cleaner house and a happier life. Yes, that is possible. Yet, when I look up from writing, I see that my bedroom door is locked tight from the temptations of the world. It's easy to feel strong behind my locked bedroom door. But as soon as I open it, I will have to get meals for my family, see and hear ads on TV, smell good smells, and face the problems of life that so often lead me to eat. I'm scared to death to unlock my bedroom door, let alone leave my room. I will have to pray with all my might to make it through the day. Just this one day. Surely I can adhere to my food list this one day.

I'm learning not to judge other people so harshly. Maybe their hair is greasy, their house is cluttered, or their yard is a mess. I don't know their trials, and I don't want to know. I just want to conquer mine.

Saturday, December 30, 1989
248 pounds

Yesterday I was fine till Allen took me out to dinner. Of course, I *had* to have that second piece of garlic toast, all my butter and sour cream, and some of Allen's leftover butter, too—and that tiny little cup of ice cream. Why, I *had* to have that.

How Allen must hate me, or at least pity me, when he sees me eat like that. Poor man. What is he to do? Oh, Allen, I shall try not to eat desserts in front of you or anyone else anymore. I lose all self-respect when I do. A big, fat lardo eating sweets. I hate myself then.

February 21, 1992. "Poor Allen," my eye! By this point in our marriage, I had been begging him for years to help me. I had told him literally hundreds of times exactly what I needed him to do. I begged, I pleaded, I screamed, I cried. As I write these words, I can't help aching over the lack of concern for my disease my husband showed for me for so many years. Reading about his blatant disregard for my problem hurts more than I can ever record. I had told him point-blank, "Make sure you discuss with me exactly what I will eat whenever we go out together." If he had taken one minute to do so, I would never have eaten that stupid "tiny little cup of ice cream." And why was the butter within my reach? And the garlic bread? If I couldn't have reached them, I would have been too embarrassed to ask for more. I ate them solely because they were conveniently accessible. All Allen had to do was move them to his side of the table. But, after all, he is a man. I guess that is asking too much! I am not blaming Allen for my obesity. But I am continually hurt by his seemingly uncaring attitude toward my horrible disease.

Wednesday, January 24, 1990
246 pounds

I am sick of failing. I want to succeed, if only for one short day. From 6:00 A.M. to 11:00 P.M. is only seventeen hours. Can't I keep my mouth in control for seventeen short hours? Today, I've been good (from 6:00 A.M. to 10:00 A.M.). Four hours. About one-fourth of the total time that I have to be in control today.

No one ever makes an effort to help me. I'd appreciate a little support from my family. In fact, I need a lot of support. I am going to refuse to take care of any of my responsibilities, to let them know how upsetting it is never to be able to depend on anyone. From now on, I'm thinking only of me.

Yesterday I was in control until I drove to the store to get Tyler's medicine for bronchitis. The second I gave the pharmacist the prescription, I headed for the candy counter. I bought three candy bars. I ate all three while I was waiting for Tyler's medicine. A 250-pound woman eating chocolate candy in front of the world, all the while dying inside with shame.

I go along fine, feeling strong and longing to be free from my fat shell, when suddenly, the time bomb goes off. I start shaking inside, and my brain screams, "No, no, go away, wicked food thought! Go away!"

If at that point, I would stop and take a deep breath, I'd be able to calm down and take control. But it's a battle with myself, because part of me is going crazy for that candy bar! If I think too hard, I'll talk myself out of the candy, so I purposely keep the deeper part of my brain (my conscience, if you will) shut off until it's too late.

I can't believe that one little candy bar is now fifty-five cents. Why, when I was young—no, I refuse to start using that line till I am at least in my sixties. Well, back in the 1950s and 1960s, when big, thick candy bars were only five cents, our neighborhood store sold them six for a quarter. Ahhhh, even a poor truck driver's family could scrape up one little quarter. And we did, regularly!

Mom had this little signal she would sing out whenever she wanted one of the children to go to the store for candy. I wish I could somehow sing the tune for you. It was similar to the old ditty, "Shave and a haircut—six bits!" Mom would merely let out a humming, grunting version of it, and children would come running from all over the house. We knew it always meant "Six-for-a-quarter candy bars!"

One day I was in my bedroom playing inside an empty television cabinet that held my teddy bears and dolls. I suddenly heard my mother's old, familiar melody ring out. I reared up like a horse recognizing a rattlesnake. Bam! I bumped my head hard on the inside top of the cabinet—so hard I nearly saw stars. But could a mere bump stop me? Heavens, no! I made a quick swipe at my head to check for blood as I raced to Mom to place my order. Neither rain nor sleet nor even a concussion could stop me.

After thirty-some years, all my siblings remember this. Barbara told me she can remember many instances when Mom sang the "candy" song twice a day. Barb was off to the store with a quarter tucked safely in her pocket. Twice a day! Mom often instructed Barbara to get six candy bars "and a Bubble Up for *me*." As if Mom weren't going to eat any of the candy. As if pop were not fattening.

Sometimes, Mom would quietly send Barbara to the store for the famous six. Barb was allowed one candy bar; Mom kept the rest for herself, giving strict instructions not to tell the other children about the treat.

There's even a pathetic finale to this little tale. Frequently, when we little children were all clamoring around for our share of the goods, Mother would cut the candy bars into pieces. She made a real show of it. "Now, you children can each have bites from more than one candy bar. Isn't this exciting?"

Poor Mother. She has the disease just as surely as I do. There was a less benevolent reason why she cut the candy bars into little pieces. She could pilfer sections of each candy bar, and we children would never know. I didn't realize what was going on as a child, but Barbara did. She often saw Mother putting some or all of her favorite candy bars away for herself, to eat later on. I guess Mother did the old hide-in-your-room-and-eat-candy-bars trick, just as I do.

Of course Mother was no dummy. She also ate her share of the community platter of cut-up candy bars, all the while eagerly anticipating her own carefully hoarded pieces. Believe me, I've become an expert at such games! Like mother, like daughter. Oh, dear God, please help me. This is one tradition I must not pass down to my daughters.

Thursday, January 25, 1990
246 pounds

How nice! I was in control yesterday and today. My, what a change! I want to be able to trust me again, yet I can never be too cocky or too sure of myself. Never, for the rest of my life, because I am a genuine food addict. I must be aware of whatever goes into my mouth till the day I die. However, if I finally have a thin body, the thought of a lifelong diet program will not be as depressing. It's the constant humiliation of being grotesquely obese *and* having to watch what I eat that gets to me!

I want to go to my twenty-year high school reunion. It's nip and tuck if I'll make it. I definitely won't go weighing over 175, but I might be as low as 162 on June 1, according to my Weight-Loss Goal Calendar. I would go at 162. Rah, Rah, Rah! Go, Rose, go! Lose, Rose, lose! I want to put on a rally uniform and chant it out!

Sunday, January 28, 1990
242 pounds

I am declaring a "War on Food"! I am through losing a pound a week while gaining three a month. Allen has promised his adamant support. Now, we all know he won't be perfect. He'll occasionally forget to ask me how I'm doing on my Daily Checklist. But I'm not going to assume the I'll-watch-him-like-a-hawk-and-see-if-he's-really-going-to-help-me attitude. I'm going to assume that he *will* help me. I'm going to take the initiative and talk to him each day about my progress. Soon it will be a habit for both of us. It's about time I made habit work *for* me.

Tuesday, January 30, 1990
243 pounds

Once, while thoroughly cleaning her kitchen, my mother found in one of the highest cupboards the oldest, blackest, most wizened banana you have ever seen. One of my brothers had hidden it there who knew how long ago. Evidently, he had wanted to ensure that there would be a banana available to him later in the day. He knew that if he didn't hide a banana, there would not be one left!

Obviously, he forgot about it. It makes me sad to think of that old banana. Not because it went to waste, but because my brother felt he had to hide it in order to keep it. I guess we should have spent a few more of our quarters on fruit, instead of candy bars.

Wednesday, January 31, 1990
240 pounds

Overeating is a sin! *Funk & Wagnalls Dictionary* defines *sin* as "a fault or error," and obesity definitely falls into both categories. John Wesley's mother said, " . . . whatever increases the authority of your body over your mind—that thing, to you, is sin." To me, sin is deliberately doing anything to our fellow beings that we know will hurt them, either physically, emotionally, or spiritually. Since I'm everyone else's "fellowman," I am also capable of sinning against me. Medical studies *prove* that obesity results in lower life expectancy, heart problems, strokes, and diabetes. Surely it is a sin to purposely inflict such wounds on my own body.

If it were possible for obesity to affect only the overeater, it would not be so grievous. But like the alcoholic or drug addict, an obese person acutely affects the lives of all who love him, care for him, or even casually observe him. My family agrees when I say that obesity has shut more doors on our family's ability to have fun than any lack of money ever has; that obesity has been the catalyst sparking more cruel words, more undeserved slaps, more tantrums, and more tense moments than any other problem in our home; that feeding my habit has sucked up more already scarce funds than any other avoidable expense.

Jesus Christ referred to His body as a temple. Can any of us feel justified in defiling our bodies, our temples, by putting such an excess of food into our mouths that it manifests itself as ugly double chins, flabby arms, bulbous posteriors, and hideous, red stretch marks?

There are many wonderful fat people. But they are, nevertheless, out of control in this area of their lives. They would be even more wonderful if they had control of their physical appetites.

Thursday, February 1, 1990
240 pounds

Jeremy volunteered me as a chaperon for his high-school band's field trip to Reno the end of March. I could weigh 210 by then, and that's almost humanish for me.

My hope level is high. I want thinness more than I've ever wanted anything in my whole life. I want to be thin *more* than I want to deliver that baby only moments before it's born. My whole heart and soul and hope for the future are wrapped up in my desire to be thin, to be someone, to be me again.

Tuesday, February 13, 1990
245 pounds

I am sick of the constant impulses to eat. All day, every day, the impulses keep badgering me like piranhas going after their prey. I must fill my mind with more important, more inspiring ideas. I must squelch that unbidden "Ah! What

goody could I make?'' thought. I must smother the
''Mmmmm, wouldn't a McMuffin be delicious right now, as
I am driving right past McDonald's?'' idea before it has a
chance to blossom . . . or to make me blossom. (McMuffin!
What a *dumb* name. But they make it sound so cute, so
McEatable.)

I am sick of those constant thoughts. I have to learn to
ignore them. I must have a reason-to-diet inspirational
thought on the tip of my tongue, immediately ready to replace
the seductive thought of food. I have no choice. I must be
mentally prepared, or the ugly face of fat will be forever
staring back at me from the mirror.

If only I had practiced a tiny bit of self-control about what
went into my mouth as a child. But I was inadvertently taught
that treats cured every ''ouch,'' candy soothed every hurt
feeling. And if one cookie made you feel good, five made
you delirious with joy!

If you want to witness total, 100 percent lack of control,
come with me on a childhood excursion to the movies. The
movies. Now, there's a place to really pig out. It's dark. You
feel completely safe opening and eating as many candy bars
as time will allow. And that is exactly what I did as a child.
I find myself shaking my head even as I write this. How
could we Linds do it to our own stomachs?

When we would go to summer matinee movies, my sister
Rebecca would buy ten boxes of Flicks chocolate drops. She
would eat every last one. She made it clear that they were
hers: she alone bought them, she alone would eat them. Ten
boxes—for a single feature!

I am mortified to admit that I also bought ten candy bars for
a single feature. I recall carefully analyzing this horrendous
amount of chocolate in my hands, mentally measuring how
long each bar would last. I had to have enough for the whole
movie. The *whole* movie! Yup, folks, that's what limited my
chocolate intake, not the fact that I was eating too much
sickening fat and sugar, but the fact that the movie had an
end. I wanted something sweet in my mouth through the
entire film.

I shudder to think of that now, yet I never sit through a film as an adult without my mouth watering for some chocolate. I think of it almost constantly, from the moment the lights first dim. There in the back of my mind, like a dormant volcano, that memory, that desire, sits. It smolders a little, it spews forth smoke from time to time, and then . . . full-blown eruption. I can't concentrate on the movie. I think of possible ways to get out and sneak some candy. I begin to hate Allen, who sits there totally oblivious of my growing desire, totally free of the compulsion for a candy bar.

> *October 4, 1991. Last night, I was reminiscing with Barbara and Rebecca about this very issue. We were laughing about our childhood moviegoing practices. Among the three of us, there has to be at least 200 pounds of extra fat. And we were laughing about still craving enough candy in a movie to have something in our mouths from curtain opening to closing. What's the problem here? Are all members of my family afraid they will somehow lose their eyesight and hearing in a theater if they are not moving their jaws?*
>
> *Barbara said she remembers bringing Jujubes to chew on as long-lasting fillers. Of course, she would bring a couple of good chocolate concoctions, too. But they went so fast.*
>
> *Rebecca confided, "All right, I'm going to tell you something, and [smiling at me] you can quote me on this. A half pound of peanut M&M's will last through a single feature. You put two at a time in your mouth and suck on them till the chocolate candy coating dissolves. You chew the peanuts, then pop in two more. Now if you go to a double feature, you will need a whole pound of peanut M&M's. And it really is preferable to bring a three-quarter-pound bag for a single feature. Then you're sure to have candy till the end of the movie. A pound will last through a double feature because*

*you can't help slowing down toward the end of a
pound of chocolates . . . and by then you are so
sick that you swear you will never do that again!''*

Wednesday, February 14, 1990
245 pounds

I keep thinking of the clothes I will have to wear in two short
weeks. My closet is full of them, full of clothes I can't fit
into. But if I remove them from my closet, it's as if I'm
giving up hope, as if I'm acknowledging I'll always be this
fat. So I leave them in there as a sign to me that someday I
might make it.

The past few days have been particularly sweet between
Allen and me. I love him deeply. I am lucky. This time, he
is trying extra hard to help me stay on my diet. Everything
is fantastic between us right now.

Sometimes, marriage seems like a roller-coaster. The highs
are so high, and the lows are so low, and it seems that one
stupid slipup can put me in the pits so fast. I am convinced
that marriage is the ultimate test in this life. If I want to pass
this test with flying colors, I'm going to have to color me
thin, first! If something bad happens in the future, even if—
gasp—Allen and I have, shall we say, a little tiff, I am going
to try to make myself remember that I can be happy. No
matter what the children, or Allen, or a schoolteacher, or a
church member does, I, Rosemary Green, can still be happy.
Things and people can't make me happy. Only I can do that.

Thursday, February 15, 1990
240 pounds

At this moment, I don't care if I'm fat forever! Right now,
I want to indulge in tons and tons of thick, sweet, fattening,
gooey stuff. ''Deep breath, slap yourself across the face,

Rosemary! Get a grip. Calm yourself down. Take another breath.'' Okay, I want to be thin more than I want to eat. The less I eat, the more I lose.

I'm proud I fought the almost uncontrollable urge to whip up a batch of yummy cookies. Thank goodness I had the strength to get out of the kitchen. What a poor, sick mess I am in; but at least I got out. (I told Allen how I had to leave the kitchen to retain any semblance of control. He immediately responded, with a silly grin on his face, ''If you can't take the treat, get out of the kitchen.'' Oh! Isn't he clever!)

I love a sign I recently saw: NOTHING TASTES AS GOOD AS BEING THIN FEELS. Monumental thought! But it's on the cupboard door of a very fat woman's kitchen. Evidently, it won't provide the magic cure I have been looking for, but I like it anyway. I'm too chagrined to put it up in my kitchen, though, in plain sight of everyone. Maybe, when I weigh 125 pounds, I'll have it printed in gold calligraphy and put on my refrigerator door to remind me of my struggle. Jenny says that when I weigh 125 pounds, I'll wallpaper the whole kitchen with it!

Friday, February 16, 1990
240 pounds

Often, at the end of a day of serious dieting, I have found myself in the kitchen, cramming food into my mouth. Anything munchable! I eat the good and the bad and then I become the ugly! The next morning, I start in where I left off the night before. Within moments of consciousness, within seconds of my eyes fluttering open, there I am in front of the fridge—sniffing, poking, searching, cramming. But this morning I was strong. I did not dash for the kitchen. If I can stay in control a few weeks longer, then habit will start working for me.

I have discovered a time when calories don't count. I wake

up in the middle of the night. What do I do? Eat, of course! I've already completed my food list from the day before. But now it is "the next day." While no one is around, I carefully, quietly eat any leftover sweets, ice cream, sandwiches, spoonfuls of peanut butter, anything chewable, then cleverly clean up after myself. Of course, everyone else is in bed, so no one ever knows. Then I sneakily put a dot of toothpaste on my tongue and swish it over my teeth, so Allen can't smell chocolate on my breath when I crawl (roll) back between the sheets.

The wonderful part of eating in the middle of the night is that, as I said before, *calories don't count*. After all, I will get up and weigh myself later, when I officially arise for the day. No use writing down on today's food list what I ate before I weighed myself this morning, because it's already on my body. I don't write it down on yesterday's food list, because as the song says, "yesterday is past and gone." So you see, since it's not written down anywhere, whatever I ate during those "magic" hours has no caloric effect on me.

Monday, February 19, 1990
241 pounds

I wore a new dress yesterday. When I say new, I really mean I haven't worn it for months because I was too fat. It's one of those rewards along the way that help keep one dieting!

Had to chuckle at myself just now. I'd gone into the kitchen to get my breakfast. Thought about a banana. According to my calorie counter, bananas have about eighty calories. The funny part is this: I don't reach for the smallest, I reach for the largest. Bananas have eighty calories, right? I might as well have the largest for the same eighty calories. It's just one of the many games fat people play. In reality, the bigger the banana, the more calories it contains. But I stupidly kid myself by choosing the biggest, while thinking, "Super! The counter says only eighty calories." What a fool. The less I eat, the more I lose! *I choose to lose!* I will eat less. I will choose the smaller piece!

It has been ingrained in me to choose the largest, most frosting-slathered piece of anything. I was trained from infancy to eat that way. We had few rules of etiquette where food was concerned. Eating was a rather unconventional experience around our home. We even had birthday cakes that threatened to self-destruct the next day: whether we made it from scratch or bought it at the store, if it was a birthday cake, Mom said all of it *had* to be eaten on the birthday.

When I was little, I used to wonder what would happen if, just once, by some miracle, there was a tiny piece of leftover birthday cake in my home. Would it decay into mush by morning?

When I was older, I understood the rationalization behind such a ridiculous policy. My family wanted to have an excuse to eat the whole cake at once, and I went happily right along with them.

Monday, February 26, 1990
238 pounds

Sometimes, the thought of mixing up a batch of cookies comes like a bolt of lightning through my mind. Lately, I've worked on quickly acknowledging that urge. Instead of nurturing the dirty thought of making those cookies, I quickly confess it. I put it out in the open so everyone knows. I don't—as I used to do—secretly hug the thought to me and wait for my chance to be alone to mix up the dough. Sometimes, I take a hurried leave of the kitchen with an "I have to get out of here." Or, I promptly tell Allen how I'm feeling, so he can help me resist.

Although I have failed miserably at many things, many times, this time I refuse to lose! I refuse to lose anything but weight, that is. I keep thinking of summer vacation (diet like crazy, girl!). My twenty-year class reunion (lose, Rosie, lose). A Green family reunion in July (I can do it). A Lutz family reunion in August (I could weigh what I did when I was married!). But most of all, I keep thinking of the rest of my life, of the important things I can do and change because I won't be "an old, fat broad."

Wednesday, March 28, 1990
232 pounds

I'm down seven pounds in two days. I think it's because of all the tears I cried yesterday. I was depressed and angry and frustrated. But repentance is a marvelous cure and a soothing balm for the burning soul. It reminds me of putting ice on a burned finger. It brings instant relief. Yet take the ice away before the burn is healed, and it keeps on hurting. I am not ever insincere when I try to repent of my sin of overeating. Each time, I believe I will succeed. Yet foolishly, I interrupt the full repentance process (which, for me, is my Daily Checklist) and fall back into my bad, old habits.

Today, I will fight back at this black depression. Hope has replaced the despair of yesterday. Of course, new problems will arise, but I don't have to get depressed and suicidal over them; I have to stand tall and meet them and work them out the best I can, and then go on with my life! Enduring to the end is more than a cliché. It is everything. I must endure to the end to win this battle with butter.

Wednesday, April 18, 1990
237 pounds

Easter. That glorious time of year celebrating the resurrection of Christ. New flowers, new buds, new life, new hope. So what do I do? Stuff my face with new, chocolate Easter candy. Oh! "My kingdom for a Rolaids!" And wouldn't you know it? I gave the last one to Allen a few days ago. Ah, well, I deserve to suffer.

I feel like a pig at this moment. Egad! I just remembered a funny-at-the-time experience from my childhood that foreshadowed all too accurately the reality that was to be. I'm not sure which one of my brothers or sisters started it, but it became a regular occurrence whenever Mother made pancakes or French toast. Because there were many mouths to feed, cooking either of those two dishes seemed to take forever. While we were waiting for our plates to be filled, we would sing the following, almost prophetic, little ditty: "We are piggies standing in line! We are piggies standing in line!" Over and over we would chant it. And we would, indeed, stand in line, ever holding out our plates for more. "We are piggies standing in line!" It's tragic how that innocent child's play set the stage for our futures.

Tuesday, May 1, 1990
242 pounds

Happy May Day! May I never weigh 242 pounds again. May I stay faithful to my diet today. May dieting be a part of my life . . . for the rest of my life. May my terrific mood of this moment be with me always. May my days be merry and bright. May all my Christmases be . . . LITE!! (Hey! I said I was in a terrific mood!)

Thursday, May 3, 1990
252 pounds

Today, I am facing reality. Today, I must put down in black and white that the scale I have been using is registering at least ten pounds low. What seems to be a ten-pound gain from two days ago is really due to the fact that I am using a different scale. Yuck! Now every record of my weight must have ten pounds of ugly fat added to it.

The last two times I have been in doctors' offices with my children, I have weighed myself. Boo and hiss. That is how I discovered that I weigh at least ten pounds more than I thought. I wish I could say that hospital scales are not necessarily more accurate, but I'm smarter than that. I must face the ugly reality that I once weighed 282 pounds (not 272) when I wasn't even pregnant. I also have come to grips with the fact that I must lose an additional ten pounds to reach my goal of 125. But I will not let it throw me into a fit of depression. I will, instead, determine to fight all the harder.

Nothing is as important as gaining control of myself. As important as putting this deadly disease out of my life. As important as reaching my full potential, or at least trying to reach it. As important as my getting thin. I am through being taken for granted. I am through being disappointed and hurt by those I love and do so much for. *I am fighting back!* Till I get well, *I'm* the most important person around here.

I must once again reiterate a principle critical to the success of my program. I am sorry to say that I have thus far been unable to adhere to it: I must take time for me. I've said it before, but I've never *done* it before! I'm even going to do more than take time for me, I am going to do a little nurturing of me. I am going to put ol' number one first for a change. Yes, that's exactly what I am going to do! I'm going to put me first, and, thus, the change will come. Me first—for a change!

I am firmly convinced that the only way I can truly diet is to adopt a whole new way of living. It takes time to diet. One has to plan and scheme and hope and dream of a future thin self. Every day. Not a short burst for a couple of days or weeks or months. I am as positive as one can be of this fundamental concept: I will have to be on a diet for the rest of my life. Everyone with a weight problem will have to do the same. It boils down to the need to endure to the end.

I've made numerous entries over the years, when I have been superhigh on my diet, to the effect that "This is it for me. I will never again have to lose those same, ugly pounds. I will never gain this weight back; I will weigh 125 by Christmas." Yet here I am again, weighing 252 pounds. To quote Joan of Arc, "But I am wiser now, and nobody is any worse for being wiser." I am much wiser. (It is the one, solitary benefit I have found that comes with age.) I now know that overeating is an addiction similar to alcoholism. "Hello, I'm Rosemary. . . . I'm a foodaholic."

Those words are not meant as a joke. I am sincere. I *am* Rosemary. I *am* a foodaholic. I will be for the rest of my life. But—and this is all-important—I can control my problem, my sickness, my disease. With the help of God, and *only* with His help, I can overcome this hideous malady.

I look at Oprah, every fat lady's heroine, and almost tremble with fear. She did it. She finally reached her dream size. She wore her famous Calvin Klein size-ten jeans on her show. And then one, two, three pounds. (No, Oprah, stop! Get back in control.) And now, eighteen pounds gained back. How far will she go? I cannot let that happen to me.

Friday, May 4, 1990
252 pounds

I've been good today. I should feel grand, but I don't. There's no eloquent or clever way to say it. I feel awful. I feel depression creeping over me. I feel it so acutely that, for the first time, I know depression is a real, tangible presence. It's more than a feeling, it's a presence! Oh great, now I'm in serious trouble. Because one thing's for sure: this is definitely not a kind, good, or holy presence. As I write this, I feel the gloom settling dramatically around me, like a thick fog. I'm a little scared.

I am proud of myself for not succumbing to this hideous feeling. I am not eating or screaming or sulking or crying. I marched into my room and opened my workbook. I am fighting back. Depression may yet hit me stronger than it has this night, but I will never again allow it to turn me into a moping, sulking fool.

Saturday, May 5, 1990
250 pounds

I feel strong today. I feel in control. And yet . . . I've felt in control before. But this time, I think I might make it . . . because I know I might not.

Today, I bought a Twix candy bar for Tyler, a dangerous thing to do! It became warm and soft in the car and was too messy for Tyler to eat the second half. When I came home, I put the leftover, squishy half in the freezer. Not for one second was I tempted.

But I am being wary about my diet. I am peeking around corners. I am waiting for the old cravings to attack me with their deadly little spears of desire, of ''but-I-deserve-just-one-little-bite-itis''! So before the enemy could attack, I built up my defenses. I erected the walls of my fortress. I set out booby traps. What I actually did was tell Allen I had put half a Twix candy bar in the freezer, and he'd better make sure it was there later, and was welcome to it.

I was proud of myself for not getting a candy bar for me when I bought one for Tyler. I was proud of myself for not eating that soft, warm, luscious, extra half that would have melted in my mouth with pure pleasure. I was proud of myself for thinking ahead to a possible mishap by telling Allen where I'd put the candy bar. But most of all, I was relieved to find the Twix candy bar gone when I opened the freezer to look for it several hours and numerous traumas later.

Sunday, May 6, 1990
249 pounds

Oh, the opposite of misery! Haven't felt like this for . . . I don't think I've *ever* felt like this. Oscar Hammerstein II knew how I feel when he wrote, "I'm . . . as high as a flag on the Fourth of July." I've been excited before, but this time I have a much more complete outline of my future in mind, so I feel that it's not some temporary, short-lived spurt of gusto. I have a chance to make it this time, because I have a much more realistic view of my weaknesses and eating habits.

I feel as if I'm walking across a frozen lake. I'm aware that the ice is thin in spots. I must be cautious about my every step. There is only one safe path across; I must not let myself get sidetracked. I must keep my eyes ever open for danger, or I will fall through and drown. My glorious goal is the far shore, where I see flowers and rainbows and Ferris wheels and fireworks and happiness. I must never lose sight of the far shore.

Monday, May 7, 1990
245 pounds

What a jerk I was last night. How ashamed I am. I wasn't even angry or depressed. In fact, I was feeling high because I had exhibited amazing self-control on my diet the past few days. Allen and I were discussing the family potluck held at my nephew Jeff's house. Jeff's wife, Christy, had commented on my pretty dress. I laughingly told Allen that I had replied to Christy, "Thank you, but I know I look like a pup tent in it."

Allen responded, "Oh, you didn't have to say that."

Snap! Something broke inside me. "I'll say what I want to say. I'm an adult. Just bug off!" Being on my diet for a few days cannot erase the years and years of hurt and agony

I have suffered. My obesity has resulted in some overly tender sensitivities. Poor Allen. I'm always on the defense. I twist and turn everything he says into something with an ugly "fat" connotation, or I take it in a negative way. I'm anxious to lose this rotten attitude along with the weight!

I admit I can't take a compliment well. Any compliments I receive about my looks cannot be 100 percent truthful. Christy was totally innocent of any offense, but she didn't mean that my dress was pretty. She probably found the material or the style attractive, but a size-twenty-four-and-a-half dress can never be "pretty." A pretty, size-twenty-four-and-a-half dress is an oxymoron. It is huge. It *is* akin to a pup tent.

What Christy would have been justified to say was, "Considering the vast amount of material needed to make that dress, and ignoring the voluminous rolls around your middle, that's a decent covering for your body." But polite people aren't that brutally honest with each other. Christy leaned toward the truth enough to say the *dress* was pretty, not that *I* looked pretty in the dress.

However, I didn't march into the kitchen and "show Allen" by eating my way from a pup tent to a four-man tent! Thank goodness for that self-control because I needed it today. Sue Land, the mother of one of my day-care children, brought us a bag of unsold food from the restaurant where she works. It contained some specialty sandwiches, a giant cookie, and a piece of cake with thick frosting. I stared at that cake for several seconds. My involuntary reflexes sprang into action. My mouth started to water. I licked my lips. I started removing the plastic wrap from the cake. I could already taste the sickeningly sweet sensation of condensed sugar, and then, *pow!* Like a ton of bricks, it hit me. "No! I want to go to my class reunion. I want to lose weight. I want to be free." I put down that blasted cake.

Today, I experienced another moment of pride. I stopped by my mother's house, and she sent home two pieces of chicken with me. Coincidentally, when I picked up Tyler from my sister Barbara's house, she also gave me two pieces of chicken to go. Four pieces of my-favorite-food-in-the-world chicken, and all for me! So where does the pride come in? I ate only one piece. *One* piece. I've never done that before in my whole life. One piece! I saved the rest for later. Yessss! I think there is hope for me yet.

Wednesday, May 9, 1990
245 pounds

Poor Debbie. Her dear little dog Mandy was killed by a car this evening. When my dog Cinnamon was killed, I was devastated. Although I don't know exactly how Debbie feels, I know how horrible it is to have your dog killed by a car.

As I drove away from Debbie's house tonight, I found myself thinking deeply about the drama of life: "Dead is so . . . dead. Life is so fragile. Emotional pain is incredibly intense. But day-to-day living still must go on. Work to do, meals to cook, weight to lose." Yes, I actually thought that. Weight to lose. Amazing.

Usually, when a tragedy strikes, it is like the red flag being waved before a bull. That flag, in big, bold letters, proclaims: THIS IS JUSTIFICATION TO EAT. YOU NEED, YOU DESERVE, THE COMFORT AND SOLACE OF FRIENDLY FOOD. Like a bull, I charge ahead, almost snorting toward my favorite candy store. But not this time. This time I thought: "Life must go on . . . weight to lose."

Thursday, May 10, 1990
243 pounds

Glorious morning! Can anything be half as exhilarating as setting goals and keeping them? I mean self-improvement, change-your-whole-lifestyle goals. No, nothing compares to it. For seven whole days, I've checked every square on my list. It feels so good to feel good.

I was sorry to hear that my parents' neighbor lost his wife a few weeks ago. But I felt especially blessed when he generously gave me many of her beautiful clothes. Not only were they my favorite colors, they were the most flattering styles for me. What a thrill to have stylish and pretty clothes to wear, even to work in around the house. I had been wearing ugly old rags—and hating it!

There are two reasons I had no decent clothes. One, we are devastatingly broke at the moment. Two, it's a nightmare to go clothes shopping when a size twenty-four-and-a-half is small on me. A horrible nightmare!

Picture it: There I am—desperately looking for the perfect dress. You know, the one that will make me look fifty pounds thinner. Suddenly, a beam of light seems to come from the heavens and illuminate it: the Thinning Dress. It's gorgeous. I'll look like a dream in it. If only it's big enough. Let's see . . . yessss! It's a size twenty-six-and-a-half. It should fit. Just look at that darling little belted waist. Oh, please, let it look as good on me as it does draping elegantly on the hanger.

I joyously go into the dressing room, almost dancing. I hang up my "perfect dress," my eyes caressing it one last time before I undo the cute little belt. And that is *my* undoing, too!

Volumes of material burst out the instant that belt is loosened. My cute, sexy, waisted dress becomes a protective covering for an armored tank. The folds just keep unfolding. I barely have the courage to try it on. Oh, gag! I *look* like a tank in it. I take it off fast, before the picture of my fat reflection in the mirror becomes indelibly etched into my brain.

I feel fatter than ever. I hate shopping. I hate the dress. I hate life. I hate Allen at that moment, and he's not even there! I detest me. I can barely leave the dressing room without bawling. I can scarcely stumble out of the store and get into my car without screaming. I gasp with self-inflicted pain and misery as I drive—not home or to a spa—but to a (yes, folks, you guessed it!) convenience store! I pick up dozens of goodies. (Why not? I saved a lot of money by not buying that dress.) I drive home in a fury, all the time munching away. I march into my room, lock the door, turn on the TV, and sink into the oblivion of chocolate and fantasy once more.

Being out of control in any area of life can be frustrating and depressing. I have discovered that striving for and achieving even a small degree of self-control is the most precious gift I can give myself. I mean, it even beats a ten-pound box of chocolates!

I tell you, when I lose another ninety pounds, shopping will hold the enchantment for me that Disneyland holds for a child. But for now, shopping is incredibly depressing. I could write a whole book on the absurdity of fat-lady clothes. But to be brief: shoulder pads, hip ruffles, short sleeves, belts, horizontal stripes, pedal pushers, and hem lengths that hit me in the fat of my calf—I don't need at this weight. And neither does one other person who wears size twenty or larger! (For once in the history of the world, are you listening, all you fat-girl clothes designers out there? Pay attention!)

Monday, May 14, 1990
245 pounds

Some time ago, I heard Oprah Winfrey say, "From a very young age, I knew I was destined for greatness." When I heard those words, it was like a giant light bulb clicking on in my brain. Yes! I related. I *knew* what she meant, how she felt. I had never put that kind of feeling, my nebulous impressions, into words. I'd never tried. But as she made that statement, I was flooded with memories, emotions, and explanations of past frustrations. In a matter of moments, these pieces of my life drenched me with a vision of my future, culminating with this one thought: "I, too, am destined for greatness." Though I'm not sure exactly how.

I am excited, yet scared to death. The immensity of what might be overwhelms me. But that underlying, thin thread of doubt arises from time to time as a thick rope, with a

"Who do you think you are?" Well, I'll turn that thick rope of doubt into a lasso and "round up" my own destiny. This thing is bigger than I am! (And I'm pretty big!)

Wednesday, May 16, 1990
242 pounds

The sun is shining and it's a beautiful day. But even if it were pouring down rain outside, I would see only blue skies and rainbows! Today, I weigh a mere 242 pounds! I am as low as I've been in a year. Since March 6, 1988, I've lost forty pounds. That's about one-fourth of what I needed to lose on that dreary March day of 1988. At this point, though, losing forty pounds would be over one-third of what I need to lose.

I get a kick out of Weight Watchers "diet desserts." I am on a *diet*, not an "eat-it"! I am not eating cheesecake. Or chocolate mousse. I don't deserve them. I've already had my share of such richness, such sweetness, to last the rest of my life. Seriously, I have. I must pay the price first, and then, perhaps, just maybe, I can occasionally afford the calories of desserts.

My biggest weakness during the past two weeks has been my failure to stick to my food list. My main emphasis on improving my diet program for the next week will be to stick exactly to my daily, preplanned menu. I haven't been eating too much, but often I have substituted this food for that food. I need to experience the discipline of eating what I say I'll eat, of doing what I say I'll do.

Several times in the last fifteen days, I have come face-to-face with extraordinary temptation. Many times, Sue Land has dropped off more goodies from work: brownies, cookies, carrot cake, chocolate cake, and poppy seed cake. One day, I grabbed a brownie and started to unwrap it. With trembling fingers, I nearly clawed off the plastic covering, thinking, "What would one little brownie hurt?" At that point, I think the prayer for strength I'd uttered that morning kicked into gear, and I heard a resounding "No!" scream out in my brain. I took a deep breath and thought for a second, "Why am I about to eat this?" And—sigh—I put the brownie down. After only thirty seconds, I was safe. It no longer tempted me. I believe God was with me in that moment when I needed my hands slapped.

Another day, overcome by an instantaneous urge, I had a piece of cake partway to my mouth when a bolt of willpower filled my whole being. I dropped the cake and hurriedly ran out of the kitchen. I was afraid not to. I rushed into my bedroom, listened to my day tapes for a few minutes, and returned to sanity. Then I was fine. I was strong. I laughed at that piece of cake instead of eating it.

I need to talk to myself daily: "Come on, Rose. Don't eat it. None of it is on your menu. Be strong. It's not worth it. You want to go to your reunion. You can do it." By preparing myself beforehand, I can meet *any* challenge. I should solicit help. Tell Allen, tell the children: "I can't have any of this. Help me. Sue Land brought three pizzas today. Make sure they're still all here at dinnertime." I should do whatever I have to do. I must never forget: "Hello, I'm Rosemary. I'm a foodaholic."

Thursday, May 17, 1990
242 pounds

I am putting my willpower on trial tomorrow. My first big test. I'm going with Tiffany on a Girl Scout camp-out. Girl Scout camp-outs always include s'mores, cookies, pastries, chips, homemade ice cream, midnight snacks, and every calorie-packed, high-fat treat imaginable. But I can do it. I can resist. I've already talked it over with Allen. I will bring my own food. When it's gone, I'm done eating.

Sunday, May 20, 1990
240 pounds

Went out of town with Tiffany's Brownie troop. Had a delightful time. Was perfect on my diet. As I preplanned, I ate only the food I brought. The food that the rest of the group had—the food that I had *paid* for—didn't exist for me. I ate only from my little ice chest. I even had food left when I arrived home. I want to go to my reunion. I am dying to go to my reunion!

Wednesday, May 23, 1990
238 pounds

Day twenty-one of perfection. I am sticking to my list as gum sticks to hair it has slept in. I am "using it and losing it." People are noticing. I never, *ever* want to have to lose these horrible fourteen pounds again. Losing and gaining and losing and gaining is devastating.

I hate it with a passion when a big fat woman does some pointedly "fat" thing. Today I chaperoned a field trip with Tiffany's class. Two mothers besides myself were extremely fat, and one of them proved exactly why she was.

I was humiliated to look anything like her. Here's the scene: We are all walking along. We stride past a "very French bakery." A few minutes later, I notice this very round, very double-chinned person with a sack in one hand and a "very French pastry" in the other. She proceeded to obnoxiously tear into this huge, turnover-type dessert. I was embarrassed for her. I was also *irritated* by her behavior. How dare she shame all of us fat people by her lack of self-control? Sure, I know: *she* was the one who was pigging out, not me. But it's like one of your family members doing something dumb or rude. You feel somehow responsible, as though you have to apologize or something. People lump all us fatties together. I hate it when one fat person's piggish actions degrade all fatties a little bit more. I was furious with myself for being "one of them" at that moment. Just another fat person.

Thursday, May 24, 1990
236 pounds

In twenty-one days I've lost sixteen pounds! I am souped up! I can feel a dramatic difference in my size. When I hang my arms down at my sides, I *feel* the absence of fat rolls. There are fewer lumps and bumps. And when I exercise? Wow! I put my hands on my waist, and *voilà*! There actually *is* a waist! I can feel a curve around the middle of my body. I find myself laughing in the shower, "My thighs are thinning down!" I can see and feel the difference when I wash them. It's wonderful! But there's a crazy contradiction: I *feel* so much better that it seems I must certainly *look* divine. I feel almost Jane Fonda–ish. I run to take a look in the mirror, and . . . oh, rats! I am still undeniably huge! If I stand there au naturel, I can't help laughing! I am a tank!

Monday, May 28, 1990
234 pounds

I am heavily disappointed in my family. They *all* know I'm trying valiantly to diet and do my Daily Checklist. They *all* know that my Daily Checklist is critical to my success. Yet last night, when I practically begged them to help me do my exercises, not one person offered assistance.

I asked for help for one lousy night! I hate myself for being this weak, but I needed some encouragement in doing my exercises. I was crying out to them all: "Please help me. I am a sick person. I am weak and need help taking my medicine. Show me a little caring. Help me back to health! *Love* me back to health. Please, please help me!"

Wednesday, May 30, 1990
237 pounds

Today Allen displayed the quintessential example of what I call "male-pattern brain damage." Can you believe that he absurdly said, "You're doing so well on your diet, I don't think you need to do your checklist anymore"? Right, Allen. When I use it, I lose it. Quitting my checklist would be like a diabetic telling his doctor, "I take my insulin shot every day, and my diabetes is under control. These shots work so well, and I'm feeling so good, I think I'll quit taking them!"

Unbelievable! "You're doing so well, I don't think you need to do your checklist anymore"! And that from a man who's lived with me for nineteen years. Yes, nineteen long, fat years. (Heavy on the fat!) But it is *Rosemary* who has carried this spare tire for eighteen of those nineteen years. *Rosemary* who knows the hell of a blubbery, bulgy, bouncy body. And it's *Rosemary* who must be ever wary, ever cautious, ever repeating, "Hello, I'm Rosemary. I'm a foodaholic." So, Allen, you might forget, but I will chant it all day if necessary for me to remember: "Use it and lose it. Use it and lose it. I will yet walk this earth a skinny woman!"

Friday, June 1, 1990
234 pounds

Summer is rushing speedily toward me, but I have fourteen more days to lose poundage, to bust blubber before school is out. I am going to have a memorable summer. It is true that the more I lose, the more I gain!

This month I will turn thirty-eight. I've spent exactly half of my life as a fat person. Half of my life! Nineteen years! So, as the song goes, "I've got a lot of living to do."

Sunday, June 24, 1990
220 pounds

I tasted it! Last night I *tasted* it. Freedom. And, oh! It does taste sweet. Sweet and incredible. I haven't felt like this for years! Try to imagine a turtle being free of its cumbersome shell. Think of it running and dancing and turning somersaults. That was me, yesterday. For a few brief moments, I escaped my fatty shell and turned a couple of somersaults.

I was at my cousin's fiftieth wedding anniversary. I saw relatives there that I'd never met before. It was wonderful because I was able to be me! And I liked me. She is a fun, enchanting person to be around. I haven't felt or acted like that for years.

I was bubbly and energetic. I was smiling and talking with everyone. I even called my family together and posed for a picture, without being sick inside! And I didn't have to hold Tyler in front of me! I didn't have to worry about someone being appalled by how much I ate, because I didn't eat too much. I didn't have to sneak around and finagle an opportunity to get seconds or thirds on the cheesecake with strawberry topping, because I had no cheesecake at all! It was a perfect afternoon.

After dinner, I found myself sitting with Jeremy and Jennifer and an eighteen-year-old second cousin, Joe. I said I thought his dad was pretty terrific for putting on this anniversary celebration for Joe's grandparents single-handedly. I was not ready for Joe's response. "Oh, my dad can be a pretty nice guy, but I have a hard time getting along with him."

Now, that is not a surprising comment coming from an eighteen-year-old young man in this day and age. But the light, fun tone of our conversation changed radically in that instant. I tried not to bawl him out, but at the same time, I wanted him to realize more clearly what his place as a "young whippersnapper" really was. I'm usually able to communicate well with young people. Probably because I vividly remember the things I disliked or that frustrated me when I was a teenager.

I explained my feelings to him, and encouraged him to think of their relationship from his father's point of view. It was an intense conversation.

When our discussion had dwindled to chitchat, an uncle who had been listening came up to me and said, "You should be on the Oprah Winfrey show. Some of your ideas are truly profound. Why, you could save America!" And he was in earnest! He said it several times. I was flattered. I loved it.

It was a monumental moment for me for two reasons: (1) Who doesn't love sincere compliments? (2) I'd been able to be *me*. To express my feelings openly without being strapped by thirty-two extra pounds. Those missing thirty-two pounds allowed me to feel alive and worthwhile and productive again.

As we were getting ready to leave the reception, my crazy dad asked my family to sing a song before we left. He was obviously proud of his five grandchildren. What the heck, there was no one at this reception but relatives. So Allen, Jeremy, Jenny, Matt, Tiffany, and I sang "You Are My Sunshine."

I am the musical weak link in our family, but I smiled a lot to make up for it. Now, you must understand, I could *never* have stood (let alone sung) in front of a group of people thirty-two pounds ago. But at 220, I felt kinda cute.

We said our good-byes and left. As we were walking to our van, Jeremy put his arm around me and chuckled in my ear, "So, are we feeling thin and cute today? Are we coming out of our fat little shell?"

"Really, Jeremy, was I that different?"

"Gee whiz, Mom, I've never seen you like that before. You were fun . . . and crazy. And I liked you that way."

Fun and crazy I *might* have been, but *me* I most definitely was. The spell continued. On the sidewalk by the van, for some reason Jeremy and I broke into a darling old song, "I've made up a game called matchin' kisses. . . ." Several years ago, Jennifer and Jeremy had performed that song, with choreography, for a talent show. Well, recalling most of the actions, Jeremy and I entertained right there on the sidewalk!

I repeat, my crazy dad . . . he opens his wallet and says, "I'll give you twenty dollars if you go back in the house and sing that song, too." Hey, people, twenty bucks is twenty bucks. Jeremy and I grabbed hands, snatched that twenty-dollar bill, and raced back to the house. We were both laughing so hard, I don't know if anyone understood our explanation: "We are earning twenty dollars—the equivalent of twelve hundred dollars an hour. No one has to listen; we just have to sing." So, choreography and all, I did it. *Me*. The real Rosemary Green. (Oh! Will the real Rosemary Green please stay alive and well?) It was ridiculously fun. I loved it. Performing is in my blood—once I get the chocolate out of it.

That was the best day of my life in years and years and years! And that without chocolate, pastries, or cheesecake topped with strawberries.

Saturday, June 30, 1990
218 pounds

Much is happening. It seems fat people sit around and think up bizarre things to do in front of me just so I'll have something to write about.

Remember my sister Rebecca? Five years ago, she was popping half-pound bags of M&M's and giant candy bars daily. She was telephoning orders for extra Girl Scout cookies—but only if I'd deliver them instantly. Remember how I felt sorry for her then, because I was *on* my diet that January through May of 1985? Only two years later, April 22, 1987, I recorded how I hated her, all 117 pounds of her. I hated her because I was *off* my diet (up to 300-plus when pregnant in 1986), and she looked like somebody's dream date: flat stomach, shapely hips, and all! She looked fresh out of high school.

Oh, Rebecca, what happened since then? When did the desire for M&M's and ice cream and fast foods again take over your soul, and now your body? You're as big as ever! I've never reached my final weight-loss goal, but you did. Tell me what happened, because I don't want it to happen to me. Elizabeth Taylor, Oprah Winfrey, and now Rebecca. I'm scared. I want to weigh 125. But if—no, *when*—I get there, how do I stay? It's terrifying. Three beautiful women who were all obese. Then all trim. Two are obese again, with Oprah climbing higher. *Stop.* Somehow, I must be different.

I have accepted this fact: *I will have to be on a diet for the rest of my life!* I want to ask Rebecca what happened. What could possibly have tasted good enough to entice her out of her size-five dress? What food was tempting enough to make her lose her waist, her looks, her pride? But I can't ask. It's too embarrassing. She hasn't said a word about my weight loss, and I haven't even raised my eyebrows about her gain. It's there before us, big as life. But nary a word is uttered.

When Rebecca stopped by a few days ago, she stepped out of her car with a box of Weight Watchers ice cream bars. Okay, now I will tell you one of the things about Weight Watchers desserts that just kills me. The Weight Watchers name has given many fat people the green light to eat. If it says Weight Watchers, cram it in. Rebecca is a perfect example.

With a box of Weight Watchers ice cream bars tucked neatly under one arm, Rebecca sat down by me on my front porch. She offered me one. She said, "They're only a hundred and ten calories." I reached for one, thinking, "That's not too bad. I eat fudge bars that are one hundred calories." Then the question came to me. How many grams of fat? My fudge bars have no fat, but these Weight Watchers bars? Seven grams per 1.7 ounce bar! Forget it. I've learned enough about fat that those seven grams made the ice cream lose its appeal for me. I felt wholesome sitting there refusing foods that were bad for me and my diet. It was such a refreshing change for me!

Then Rebecca opened another of those slim, little Weight Watchers ice cream bars . . . and another. She offered one to Tiffany and Jeremy, who were talking with us. As she ate her fourth and fifth Weight Watchers bars, I had to struggle to choke down a laugh. Think about the contradiction here: a person worrying about her weight, eating five ice cream bars in a row. Rebecca offered Jeremy and Tiffany one more and also Matthew, who popped his head out to say hi.

I must admit, it was almost impossible to keep a straight face when Rebecca opened her sixth ice cream bar. Yikes! We were now up to 660 calories and 42 grams of fat! But she didn't stop there. She finished off that box by eating her seventh Weight Watchers ice cream bar. Weight Watchers! It just kills me. It almost screams out, "If you want to watch yourself put on some real weight, eat me!"

Then Rebecca said, "Today, I only ate seven bars. I'll be okay. When I eat all twelve, it does get a little too rich." Oh, crazy, crazy world. Can you believe it? I've talked with many people who buy Weight Watchers food products and practice the following philosophy: As long as it says Weight Watchers, you can eat all you want. My friend Emily, who lost over 100 pounds on a liquid diet, but is dangerously obese again, keeps her freezer crammed full of Weight Watchers, Lean Cuisine, and Jenny Craig foods. She eats some of those foods . . . *and* the regular dinner everyone else in her family eats, too.

Hey! There's no magic in the stuff. If you want to lose weight, you *have* to cut down your caloric intake. It's that simple. If Weight Watchers, Lean Cuisine, or Jenny Craig foods motivate you to be disciplined, great. Buy all you want. But believe me, when you buy a package of twelve Weight Watchers ice cream bars and then eat them all at once, you're only making Weight Watchers richer and yourself fatter. They're taking money off of you, not pounds!

Friday, July 6, 1990
212 pounds

I did it! I accomplished my 40/60 plan. It worked because I worked my checklist! I lost forty ugly pounds in sixty beautiful days!

I have been submerging myself in reading my diary. I spend several hours a day on it. I am constantly astonished by the misery and darkness I have gone through for so many years. I feel a frantic desperation never to have to go through that again. Never. It is too horrible; it is my worst nightmare.

Tuesday, July 17, 1990
211 pounds

Today, Matthew had a few friends over. They were talking in the front room. While working at the dining room table, I overheard their conversation. Somehow, the subject of dieting came up. One boy almost exploded with laughter about his fat sister's use of the diet drink Slim-Fast. He giggled as he quoted the popular TV advertisement, " 'Give us a week and we'll take off the weight.' Heck! She drinks a whole week's worth in one day!" All the boys hooted. I had to chuckle, myself.

Yet I understood the pitiful plight of this boy's sister. A teenage girl. In the most sensitive years of her life, part of her dying inside to be pretty and sexy and appealing. But she is at least fifty pounds overweight. Yes, I know the feeling well. She is grasping at her Slim-Fast drink as if *it* were going to make her slim. Make her slim without exercising. Make her slim without giving up fattening foods. Make her slim without paying the price. In desperation, we obese people draw some mighty stupid conclusions. I have no reason to doubt that Slim-Fast works, but *only* if used as intended— as a meal substitute. It is not a treat to be had every couple of hours.

I'm afraid fat people get their brain cells clogged with fat, too. This girl was using the quintessential, silly "fat-rationale." I could practically read her mind: "It's called Slim-Fast. The more I drink, the faster I'll get slim." I'm not kidding. We desperate fatties can rationalize drinking ten diet shakes a day with that stupid line of reasoning.

Thursday, July 26, 1990
209 pounds

I have decided to take this diet even more seriously. I want to lose twenty more pounds before my twenty-year reunion. So I am being super-duper strict till then. No eating out. No "substitutions" on my Daily Menu. I have Fruit Loops for breakfast; one cup equals 110 calories. I have Alba 77 for lunch; one serving equals 70 calories. I have a frozen dinner for—you guessed it—dinner; one serving equals 260 calories. Breakfast, lunch, and dinner. Then I carefully measure one pound of fruit or vegetables. One pound of apricots equals 217 calories. I can nibble from that measured plate all day. That's a total of 657 calories. I love it. I've done it for the last three days. Hopefully, it will be my key to losing twenty for my "twenty" in twenty-three days.

> *February 25, 1992. I did stick to that diet for several weeks. It was surprisingly easy. However, because of reading much about the danger of extremely low-calorie diets, I now always eat at least 800 calories a day.*

Monday, August 6, 1990
206 pounds

Last night, Allen and I were cracking up. It was such a fun mood. It has been exhilarating lately with me on my diet.

There is little anger or frustration floating around the house. It's an all-too-vivid documentary on the fact that my obesity, my self-hatred, has caused frequent discord in the past. I hate that thought. But I love the laughs we had last night. Allen and I can now joke about certain "fat" things that were taboo topics three short months ago.

One of the lines I am continually telling my children came up: "There are pros and cons to everything." Allen and I both know, only too well, the million and one cons to obesity. But being in a crazy mood, we came up with some pros to being fat. Here are a few examples:

Allen: "If we were at war with some medieval enemy, and we had to go into battle with those ancient, stone-slinging catapults, and one of us had to jump on one end of the catapult to make the stone on the other end fly toward the enemy, you could make the stone go farther than I could."

Me: "If we were camping during a windstorm, and we couldn't find any big rocks to hold down the tarp covering our supplies, and one of us had to be used as ballast, I could stand higher wind gusts than you."

Allen: "If you were rowdy at a party, and the bouncer was supposed to evict you, chances are he wouldn't try too hard."

Me: "If Martians came down and were somehow able to vacuum all the food off the face of the earth, I could survive longer than you."

Allen: "If you were building a high-rise out of bricks, under primitive conditions, and you had only a rope and a pulley to get the bricks to the top of the building, you could be tied to one end of the rope and raise more bricks in a single load than I could."

Me: "Two fat people sitting together in a vehicle could smuggle a skinny person 'over the border.'"

And the list continued. Well, it was late, and everything we said seemed hilarious. However, after a thorough analysis of the "pros" of obesity, the consensus was: I am still going to try to get thin . . . and pray the Martians won't attack with their food-sucking machine!

Friday, August 10, 1990
205 pounds

I have been reading *Anne Frank: The Diary of a Young Girl* this summer. I'd read it before, a million years ago, when I was a teenager. I was amazed that I have experienced many of the same feelings and frustrations Anne described. Such different circumstances, such similar feelings. Her experience of being in hiding was a wretched tragedy. There were many things she longed to do. Her activities were dramatically restricted by her circumstances—*circumstances beyond her control*.

And what about me? The real me? Oh, the real me has been in hiding these many long years. I have craved to do innumerable things, but my activities have been severely restricted by my circumstances. But here's the difference, the all important difference between Anne and me: *I am in complete control of my circumstances*.

Wednesday, August 15, 1990
205 pounds

Dear Diary, I had an overwhelming urge to write that—for you have been a dear diary, a good friend. You have listened to my every woe and to each minute success. Yet this, my greatest success, what hopefully will become known as my final battle, I have not recorded sufficiently.

Right now, as if in possession of a special gift from God, I find myself with nothing but time on my hands. I am sitting here in the Girl Scout cabin at Seaside, Oregon, all by myself. I am on a mother-daughter week with my darling Jennifer. She is swimming with her friends, and I am sitting here in complete solitude. I just finished a delicious, old-fashioned love story, *I'll Get Over It*, by Maysie Greig. (A sweet story of noble young men and virtuous young women, so unlike the filthy, trashy story lines by many of today's authors.) I have no inclination to read any more. And (sure sign from heaven) the TV does not work.

Finally, at thirty-eight years of age, I am beginning to feel in control of me. Not a flash-in-the-pan control, but a real, I'll-strive-for-the-rest-of-my-life kind of control. These past few weeks, it seems that every fat person I know has approached me and brought up dieting. I purposely keep quiet about it—unless someone else brings it up. But I guess my recent, forty-seven-pound weight loss (since May 3) has become apparent enough that others are constantly asking questions or making comments.

I want to tell you many things. The first is simple, Diary: I fit! I fit on a chair! A few weeks ago I was sitting in church, when suddenly I realized, with a burst of pure pleasure, that I don't hang over the edge of the chair anymore! When I sat down, there was a smidgeon of chair sticking out on either side of me. I wanted to stand up and cheer. I wanted to scream out, "Hey! Look, you guys! I don't bulge out over the seat of this chair anymore." I couldn't help wearing a proud, yes-I-did-it! smile on my face. Every few minutes, I would oh-so-nonchalantly put my hands on either side of the chair seat, just to make sure. And, yessss! I still fit. Oh, glorious day. Oh, wonderful moment. TO FIT!

My second story is about my Lutz family reunion and the trampoline. I jumped on it! I wouldn't have even looked at it forty-seven pounds ago. But at a mere 205 pounds, I ventured forth to fun. And I loved it. It was like experiencing another dimension. My sister Debbie came up to me and reminded me of a few months earlier, when she had jumped on a trampoline for the first time since high school. She giggled and whispered, "I *told* you it was better than sex." Well, I wouldn't go that far. . . .

My Lutz family reunion. My maternal grandparents' descendants. They had fourteen children; nine are living. Sweet people. I love them all. My aunts Delsie and Kappy always make me feel special and extremely loved. This time, they both made me feel especially pretty and much thinner. I delighted in it. I reveled in it. It was a fabulous day for me.

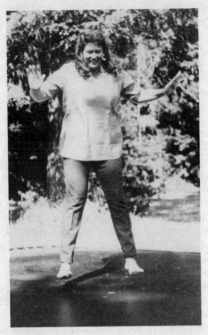

August 1990, 205 pounds. I was experiencing a delicious freedom from fat!

I even entered into a water fight with my cousin Vicky, and it was like old times. I was young again. Life was fun again. I could run again. (I think I just wrote a song!)

It was a perfect day. It was especially pleasant to be able to talk with everyone and not have to worry about looking like a tank when I sat down or like a hippo when I moved. I feel as if I've earned the right to be myself.

Just before leaving the reunion, I became involved in a conversation with two of my cousins. Lo and behold, the subject of weight came up. We discussed blubber inside out and upside down. Our jaws were moving so fast, you'd have thought we were a-goin' down on a box of fancy chocolates.

It was a most interesting conversation. One hefty cousin professed that women were supposed to get fat when they had children, as if it were part of a plan. She declared that she was never again going to diet because she always gained weight when she did. It was interesting to me that this cousin was so adamant in singing the praises of one particular "eating program" (heaven forbid I should use the word *diet*). She kept going on and on about how fantastic this program is, how easy it is to lose weight on it—yet she wasn't using it, herself.

Then my cousin proceeded to expound upon the chief reason she didn't want to lose weight: she was afraid of losing muscle. Oh, please! The "losing muscle" reason for not dieting blows me away. I'd gladly give up a little muscle if I could lose a lot of fat with it.

My cousin was furious that people judge a person by their appearance. Well, those that judge me fat are right. I *am* fat. Those that judge me unable to control myself around food are right. I *can't* control myself around food . . . or I couldn't. And sorry, dear cousin, while a pregnant woman's tummy should get fat, her upper arms and neck and thighs definitely should *not*!

There's only one reason people don't lose weight when they diet: *they don't ever really go on the diet. Any* doctor-approved diet will work *if the person will work the diet*. The whole conversation made me feel as if I were in the "Twilight Zone" and that I was *the last honest fat person in America*. I am more convinced than ever that it is extremely difficult for a fat person to honestly face the facts and face the fat!

However, my Aunt Delsie stood solidly behind my philosophy. And she is one woman whose opinion I deeply respect. She is also one woman who is quick to give her opinion. She took me aside and whispered in my ear, "Rosemary, I am thrilled you are losing weight. I have been fat all my life, and I know how hard it is to control. But you are so beautiful, and I love you so much, it has been hard for me to see you overweight. I am thankful you have done this before you turned forty. I have worried about you a great deal."

Dear Aunt Delsie. I am sorry that I caused her any worry. I wonder how many other people that care about me have been concerned about my weight. And some of the "Big Is Beautiful" promoters of today would have us believe that a fat person's weight is their concern alone!

What else is new? My conversation with a Girl Scout mom. This fat lady declared, "I don't care if I *am* fat. I'll do anything I want to, and I don't care if someone doesn't like how I look. My therapist told me I'm not that special—nobody notices me, anyway." Oh, get real! I can't believe that anyone would pay good money for that kind of preposterous advice. Fat people attract attention each and every time they go anywhere. They are pointed out and laughed at. And believe me, no one is saying, "Oh, I want to look like that 300-pound woman when I grow up!"

Paradoxically, she bragged about her new diet, how much she'd lost, how easy it was. I'd known her for months but couldn't detect one ounce of weight-loss on her ample person. People should let the diet do all the bragging. In fact, only today, I met a woman I hadn't seen for several years. I loved it when she popped open her eyes and almost gasped, "Rosemary, you look *fabulous*! You've lost a lot of weight." I didn't have to brag about my diet; my body did all the bragging for me!

Yesterday I felt as if I were in a movie. Jennifer and I were enjoying a bike ride together along the Seaside Promenade. The promenade offers two miles of the most delightful bike riding anywhere in the world, with a breathtaking view of the ocean! Not only is it paved, but no motorized vehicles are allowed along the complete length. With the sun reflecting magnificently on the white waves as they rolled in, and the cooling breeze blowing gently on us, I couldn't help feeling I was experiencing a true bit of heavenly bliss. It seemed as if the whole scene had been created exclusively for Jennifer and me, as if, at any moment, someone would yell, "Cut! That's a print!"

And then, more magnificent than the sun's reflection, more innervating than the breeze, more heavenly than the bliss, one simple word penetrated my hearing and my heart. Even if it hadn't been a handsome man who said it (but it was!), I would hold him in fond remembrance forever. As Jennifer and I turned our bikes around at the south end of the promenade, I distinctly overheard him tell his wife that we must be sisters. *Sisters!* Oh, the dear, dear man! Oh, the fine, kind gentleman! Yessss! I was thankful for every dirty, rotten pound of lard I had just lost. I rode my bike a little more snappily. I held my head a little higher. I smiled a little more broadly. Sisters! Why, I felt like I was seventeen again. It was an awesome moment. I will never forget it. Even if it was almost shattered only a few minutes later.

Oh, those blasted, awful, mirrorlike store windows! How dare they tell the truth? Just when I thought it was safe to go walking down the street without looking like the Goodyear blimp, just when I thought I was cute and seventeen and looking like a sister to my daughter. *Pow!* A store window hits me smack-dab in the reality zone. Yup, folks! All the happy thoughts, blissful moments, and complimentary words in the world can't begin to hide thirty pounds of extra lard hanging around your middle. That nasty ol' store window pointed that out. I gasped to Jennifer as we biked along, "Do I look as scary from the back as I do from the side?"

"No, your fat only pouches out in front of you. You're not that big from behind, Mom." I think that made me feel better.

Even the ugly reality of my massive stomach could not spoil that delightful day. But it did ignite a fierce fire within me. I refuse to live out the remainder of my days with such a disgusting tire of blubber hanging around my middle. I will yet walk this earth a thin woman. I will yet wear—and look good in—a waisted dress. (And, let's get real . . . I will yet have a tummy tuck!)

My summer fun actually started while I was at Rockaway

Beach a few weeks ago. Allen and I rented a Buddy-Bike, a tandem bike with seats side-by-side instead of one in front of the other. I had a ball. I felt like a real person, experiencing life at last.

We also went bowling. When you're as fat as I was forty-seven pounds ago, bowling is taboo. To expose the world so mercilessly to one's big derriere is simply out of the question.

Then I experienced crabbing. I actually put my foot, followed by my body, in this little old rowboat. It would have been impossible for me to go crabbing three months ago. I would have been horrified at the prospect of merely stepping into the boat. It must be every fat person's nightmare: you step into a boat . . . and it tips over, or worse yet, it sinks! No way! I wouldn't have taken a minute chance at that one.

Sadly, biking, bowling, and boating were out for me forty-seven pounds ago. The pain of nonparticipation is especially acute when I consider the fact that I brought this torture on myself. But no more! Do I ever relate to Dr. Martin Luther King's soul-stirring line (paraphrased), "Free at last! Free at last! Thank God Almighty, I'm free at last."

Sunday, August 19, 1990
204 pounds

My twenty-year reunion. Did I have the nerve to go? A full sixty pounds heavier than I had been in high school? I couldn't decide till the very last minute. Last second, even. I had been smart enough to cover my bases, though. Before I mailed my reservations in July, I was honest with Allen: "Honey, you have to understand one thing. The fact that I'm sending in this forty-dollar registration fee doesn't necessarily mean I will have the nerve to go. Even if I do phenomenally well on my diet this next month, I will still be very fat for the reunion on August eighteenth. You must realize that we might be wasting the forty dollars. And you can't get upset with me if that happens."

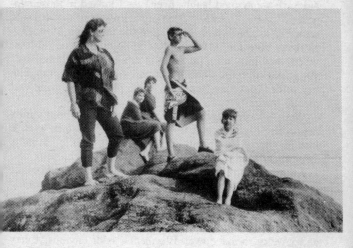

July 1990, 208 pounds. It was actually *fun* to pose for this picture with Jennifer, Matthew, Tiffany, and Tyler!

Allen was incredibly understanding: "The forty dollars doesn't matter. It's just important to me that you feel you can go." Quite frankly, the forty dollars did matter. In fact, I had to send a money order for the registration fee because our checkbook balance was so precariously low at the time that a check might have bounced if it weren't cashed at exactly the right moment.

I came home from my heavenly Seaside vacation with Jennifer late Friday afternoon. My class reunion was scheduled for the weekend.

On Friday night, I went to several different stores. Trying to lose all the weight I possibly could, I had waited till the day before my reunion to go shopping for that perfect dress. You know, the one that would make me look ten years younger and fifty pounds slimmer. Good luck, Rosie!

Needless to say, I did not find the dress. But Jenny and I

did have some good laughs over how I looked in those supposed "fat-girl" clothes. That night I resolved that I would
someday establish a clothing store for fat ladies. A *serious*
clothing store for fat ladies. Not some dumb establishment
where they hire other fat ladies to tell you how "fabulous"
you look in that size-twenty-four-and-a-half belted affair with
hip ruffles and shoulder pads. (Oh, please, spare me that
mental image!)

Well, I wasn't depressed by what could have been a truly
depressing experience. I was more determined than ever to
lose another sixty pounds superfast. Let's see . . . I had a
full twenty-four hours. . . .

Saturday morning, I had not yet decided if I could make
the final commitment. It was still too scary. I had this horrible
vision of myself hesitating in the doorway of the reception
hall. Every woman in the room was dressed as if ready to
go to the Academy Awards, with figures like Dolly Parton
and jewelry to make even Elizabeth Taylor envious. Every
hair on every head was perfectly styled and outrageously
curly and full. Every fingernail was painted and extended a
full half inch over the end of each slender finger. Every
woman wore five-inch heels and had shapely legs. Every
female had one hand gracefully resting upon her hip, while
the other hand femininely held a champagne goblet from
which the owner demurely sipped. Almost as if choreo-
graphed, every head turned as I entered, and an audible gasp
of disapproval rose up, as did one corner of every mouth,
registering disdain! With a mental picture like that, no wonder
I couldn't commit myself!

Allen assumed that we were going and told me how proud
he was to be my husband. Nevertheless, huge doubts nagged
at me throughout the day. Could I really go and expose to
all my old classmates the awful thing I had done to myself?
Could I, Madison High's 1970 Rose Festival princess, openly
acknowledge the affair I'd had with chocolate all these years?

When Allen was shaving and I was putting the finishing
touches on my makeup, I warned him, "I'm still not sure
that I can handle this." As we were going out the door, and

all the children were waving good-bye, I told them, "We might be back in a few minutes because I'm feeling extremely insecure about going."

Their "Oh, Mom, you look gorgeous!" response didn't help me decide, either. While on the way, I asked Allen, "Do I honestly want to put myself through this humiliation?"

Allen replied reassuringly, "Honey, you're going to have a super time." Upon arriving, I found myself biting my lips. I didn't *have* to get out of the car. I was an adult now. I could do whatever I wanted, and no one could ground me or anything!

"What do you think, Allen? Am I a complete fool to go in there?" He just grinned and took my arm, ushering me into the lobby of the hotel. My palms were sweaty, I was swallowing hard. It was not too late. No one had seen me yet. No one knew I was in the building. If we left now, I'd be safe. I stopped and turned to Allen, shaking slightly. "I haven't decided if I have the nerve to go in, Allen."

Dear, sweet Allen. Still my knight in shining armor. What would I ever do without him? "Honey, you're beautiful. Stop worrying."

And then . . . we were there. No going back now. Too late to retreat. But I didn't need to retreat! Ha! There was one important factor I had not taken into consideration: I was not the only person in the room who was twenty years older. Why, the room was full of pot bellies, bald heads, wrinkles, and gray hairs. And, yessss! Oh, thank you, God. Thank you, thank you, thank you! I was not the fattest person there. Not by a long shot. I actually counted, and there were at least ten people bigger than I. In fact, I quickly came to the conclusion that, what I made up for in weight, I lacked in wrinkles.

It was splendid to see old friends. With Allen by my side, I felt invincible. We strolled all over that banquet room. Most people recognized me, even before they looked at my name tag. I think that was a good sign. I didn't eat much, in spite of a lovely buffet table. And I didn't have my picture taken. After all, there was no baby to hold, and I was at this reunion by the skin of my teeth. If pictures really do put on ten pounds, I would have been in serious trouble!

The evening was incredibly fun. I learned a few things, too. No, I'm not going into some phoney dissertation, with lips quivering, about looks not mattering after all. How I looked mattered like crazy. If I had been one ounce heavier, I could never have walked into that room to begin with. I learned that, for the most part, men get sexier and women just get older. I mean, here was this roomful of virile, handsomely mature men . . . and a bunch of middle-aged women trying desperately to look as they did in high school.

I learned that if you are once a member of the "center-hall" gang, you are always a member. You know, that very elite group who congregate in a very visible place. The group you can't even say "Hi" to without a sort of understood permission. Well, they were there, big as life. And where were they parked for the night? In the *center* of the room. I'm not kidding you. And, yes, it was understood that the center of the room was their territory. And, no, I couldn't say "Hi." (But I couldn't help chuckling. And you know what? Even center-hall girls get wrinkles!)

I learned that many people remember many things about you that you don't remember about yourself. I learned that I have missed out on much more than I thought, that breaking out of the fat-jail I have been in for years is more fun than I could have dreamed. And, oh . . . yes . . . I learned that if you wear two girdles at one time, you shouldn't sit down for too long, or the top girdle will roll into a tight knot around your waist and almost cut you in half!

Thursday, September 20, 1990
204 pounds

Oh boy, was I mad this morning, and sorry and shocked and disappointed. I thought maybe Joan Rivers had learned her

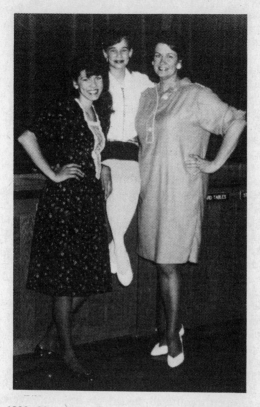

August 1990, 204 pounds. This is the dress I wore to my 20-year reunion. This picture was taken a few days after, with my two beautiful daughters, Jennifer and Tiffany.

lesson regarding Elizabeth Taylor. I thought maybe, with the tragedy of her husband's suicide, she would let up on others' problems. Shame on you, Joan Rivers. You beat up Elizabeth unmercifully. Yes, she was fat. But surely you knew she hated it. She hated her fat and the dirty rotten jokes you made about her. I repeat, shame on you, Joan Rivers!

Elizabeth Taylor showed you. In her interview with Oprah Winfrey, after she'd lost all her excess weight, she told how much the fat jokes hurt. She exposed your cruelty and the cruelty of others. During that interview, Miss Taylor looked every bit the "goddess of beauty" she ever was. My heart aches for her as I see her gain weight back, and my heart aches for me. It aches for every single fat person suffering this cursed affliction.

I was enraged with you this morning because you were degrading yet another fat person. Why can't you tell *nameless* fat-people jokes? Why do you have to single out and tell jokes about a *particular* fat person? I can appreciate a fat joke. But to single out one fat person—that's sheer cruelty. You even had a rude joke, specifically designed to hurt Delta Burke, displayed in print on the TV screen.

I didn't laugh when I saw it this morning. It will never amuse me. I noticed that your audience wasn't rolling in the aisles, either.

Delta Burke. Now there is a beautiful woman. A beautiful, overweight woman. I suffer for her as I suffer for all fat people. But I must admit, *Designing Women* is one of my favorite TV shows of all time, and her acting, her style, is very much a part of the reason. It encourages me to see her achieving success, even though she is (oh, I hate the word) fat. It inspires me to see an extremely beautiful, well-manicured, expertly coiffured, flatteringly dressed, exceptionally classy fat person. I want to be her kind of fat lady!

Today at noon, I observed twelve women waiting to pick up their morning kindergartners. Five of them were dreadfully obese. Yuck. I received the message loud and clear. Almost half of these mothers or day-care providers were obese! Being a stay-at-home woman in this day and age is dangerous. With a combination of garbage TV (soap operas, etc.); fixing children's lunches, snacks, and dinners; and all the instant puddings, pies, candies, cookies, and frozen delights available at every corner convenience store, we simply don't have a chance. Six of us had fallen to the seduction of food and were pathetically ponderous. I am determined that there will soon be one less obese mother waiting at the school!

Sunday, October 28, 1990
210 pounds

Even after my recent phenomenal weight loss, I am experiencing near torture trying to stick to my diet. Today I shall blame my eat-all-you-can-get-your-hands-on upbringing for my current struggle to maintain! Once again, I dip into my childhood memory bank. My father often brought home treats in his lunch pail. We children raced to be the first to greet Dad upon his arrival home from work. First come, first to get candy bar! Grab that pail out of his hands. Didn't matter if you were first yesterday or for the past three weeks—if you were fast enough, you secured the reward once again.

I have learned from years of experience with my own children that the candy bar in the lunch pail was as much for Dad as it was for us. I am sure there was not one time he put a candy bar in his lunch pail that he didn't put an identical one in his mouth. Stopping to get "something for the kids" was really a ploy to get "something for Roy"!

Wednesday, November 7, 1990
206 pounds

On Halloween, I bumped into Rebecca at Mom's house. Rebecca and I both laughed when I pointed to her daughter Adriane's huge pot of Halloween loot and said, "Meeep, meeep, meeep . . . red alert, red alert!" But I didn't laugh the next day at Rebecca's response to my idea of freezing some of that candy to keep it from getting stale: "It won't get stale. I'll help Addie eat it. I always put in an IOU for whatever I eat. Then she can buy fresh candy whenever she wants to.'' I didn't laugh. There was nothing to laugh at. A sob or two would have been appropriate, though, because Rebecca is now bigger than I have ever seen her.

Saturday, November 10, 1990
206 pounds

I felt free today. I stood in the open doorway of my jail and took a deep, fresh breath of air. I took several steps out into the real world. What I actually did was say hello to a friend I hadn't talked to for years, Steve Lawpaugh. I grew up next to the Lawpaugh family. We played tag, darebase, kick-the-can, merry-go-round rides, and all the fun, outdoor games lost to this generation of video addicts. We had attended grade school and high school together. The memories flooded over me. It was wonderful to recall the old, carefree days.

Allen and I talked with him for an hour. It was incredible to have had the freedom to initiate the conversation. I hadn't had to turn my eyes away and pretend I didn't see him. I hadn't had to cringe inside and die the thousand deaths, as I did a few years ago when I saw my old boyfriend in the same store.

Sunday, December 9, 1990
207 pounds

I am in the depths of misery. My soul is aching. Oh, hellish, hellish day. I don't think I can go on, this hurt and anguish is overpowering. My fingers are struggling to simply move. I'm sure I shall erase this entry, but I must tell someone how I feel. The problem is, there is no human I can talk to. I have no real friends, only acquaintances. No one knows me. No one wants to know me, and I don't blame them. I can't trust anyone with my feelings. Allen doesn't understand, or doesn't try to understand, or doesn't give a rip. Why should anyone else? I am exhausted from the struggle to be understood. Henceforth, I shall merely exist till I am released from this miserable life by my death!

Tuesday, December 18, 1990
208 pounds

Egad! Was I really that depressed? And only nine days ago! It is such a tragedy to me that I ever feel that low. Depression is a vicious creature. It breeds on itself like a monster from some outer-space movie. It's horrifying. Since last May, I have not been depressed for any significant length of time. December 9 was my lowest point emotionally in eight months. And thank you, no! I don't care to go down there amidst the misery, pain, and the devil himself again.

Sometimes I feel myself falling into the deep well of despair. I try to stretch out my arms and legs as far as they will reach, in order to claw the sides of the walls and stop my descent to hell. The reason I have not suffered such severe depression these past months is simply because I have kept a semblance of control in my life. But September through December have been nowhere near as elating as May through August. I was riding high last summer. And why? Because I was in control. *I was in control of me!* I want to be there again. My blood is once again churning with hope and desire to succeed, churning with determination to make something of myself (something less of myself)!

Sunday, December 30, 1990
213 pounds

New day. New week. Almost new month. Close to new year. What better time to put my life in order again? Why wait till I've gained back every hideous pound of blubber? If I dig in my heels, I'll have to lose only ten of those pounds over again. That's right, folks, I'm up ten frightful pounds since October 13. I can feel it. I can see it. I can touch it. I can hate it!

Everyone else can see it, too. Last night at our annual Lind family Christmas gathering, no one told me how good I was looking. No one asked me how much more weight I'd lost. Why not? Because they knew I was up a few pounds.

Food has made my body ten pounds uglier, my nights uncomfortable, my clothes too tight, and my stomach feel constantly bloated like an overblown balloon ready to pop! No, that is not true. Let me rephrase that sentence. Food has not made me experience any of that. I have voluntarily allowed food—the enemy—to invade my body, my life, and do the damage. I must not forget that it is I, and only I, who willingly opens the door. Gee whiz, for the last few weeks, I have flung wide the double doors. I have laid down the welcome mat, rolled out the red carpet, put up signs announcing, "This is the place. All candies, cookies, fudge, brownies, sandwiches with cream cheese and heavy mayo, ice cream, pastries, and anything else with over 100 calories per bite . . . come on down!"

Rip! Thwing! Yank! Bang! Did you hear it? Well, folks, I did it. I tore up those nasty ol' signs, rolled *up* the red carpet, took *in* the welcome mat, and slammed those doors tight. Now listen to this: *Scrape, click, rattle rattle!* I bolted those double doors, locked them shut, and drew a huge chain across them. Any sweet thing that gets past my security system will be so mangled and unappetizing, it will never be worth the calories.

So—deep breath—today, I will make the effort. Tomorrow, I will be thinner . . . and happier. So will my poor family, my poor, dear Allen.

Back to last night. Remember how I said no one told me how good I was looking? Well, partly it was because I'm not looking too good. But it was also because it's hard to bring yourself to compliment someone's weight loss if you have recently gained several pounds yourself! Looking at my family, it was obvious that I was not the only one who had gained a few pounds in the past several weeks. Now, I said that as sweetly as possible. We are one *big* family. And I don't mean just in numbers. I am trying desperately to break this cycle of obesity.

I had promised my children and Allen that I would not eat one sweet thing last night at the Lind family gathering. The fact that I brought up the subject shows I wanted to control my eating. It shows that I was struggling. It was my way of pleading for help. I am not angry, but if only one member of my family had stayed by my side, showed me they cared, reminded me of my commitment, I could have come home from that family gathering proud of myself. Why doesn't anyone regard my obesity as the sickness it is? Why do my children and husband make me walk this miserable road alone? When they are sick, I take them to the doctor. When will someone try to understand and help me?

I have strayed from my subject. Back to the Lind family gathering. I stayed near the food in the kitchen most of the night because that's where nearly everyone was. In the kitchen. Yikes! Is there a message here, or what?

Thankfully, I showed *some* self-control. I kept repeating to myself, "It will be gone in the morning. Whatever I eat tonight, the taste will be gone in the morning." Yet I still ate too much. And the taste *is* gone, but not the calories. Not the fatty globules. Not the shame. My only comfort is knowing I've done worse in the past.

I worry about the children. I saw my nieces—skinny, beautiful little creatures—sitting on chairs directly in front of the food table, their plates piled high with nothing but desserts. Nothing but desserts because that's almost all that was brought to the family gathering. Skinny, beautiful little girls. Do they even have a chance at staying that way?

Once again, last night, I determined that I will at least give *my* skinny, beautiful daughters a chance. I will get control of me. I will break the vicious chain of heredity and environment.

A few days ago, I watched Sally Jessy Raphael. She seems

to be a kind person. Her guests were couples who were experiencing difficulties in their marriages because of a partner's weight loss. It was interesting. (Ha! As I typed that last sentence, a mental picture flooded my mind. I was back in my kitchen watching Sally's show on weight loss . . . while baking chocolate chip cookies! That's the story of my life!)

During this program there were some unusually honest comments made about obesity. At the end of the show, Sally took the mike to a sister of one of the lady guests who had lost weight.

Sally: "As the sister of an overweight person, how do you feel about all this?"

Sister: "I'm the thin one in the family. I always have been. I wish that people would forget about weight and get on with their lives."

Big applause from the audience. Like the sister had said something profound. "Forget about weight and get on with your life." To some people I'm sure that sounded realistic, even clever. I wanted to scream out to the audience, "But don't you see? Don't you get it? Obesity prevents one from getting on with life. Obesity keeps a person from the kind of life he wants. Almost *all* physical activity is out of reach of the fat person. Please tell me how one goes about 'getting on with life' when one can't even get *into* one's jeans?" We obese people must continue our day-to-day living; we have no choice. But we can't forget about our weight. It is a noose around our necks and the rest of our bodies—an ugly, fatty, fleshy noose!

Friday, January 11, 1991
212 pounds

Am I waging a personal vendetta against Joan Rivers? I don't think so. In fact, I admit she is a talented lady. When she's not being obnoxiously obscene, she can be hilarious. I don't watch her show often, but each time I do, she maligns some overweight person. Today I was gratified to hear that her viewers are not particularly thrilled with her scathing remarks, either. She had asked her viewers to phone in and respond to the question of whether she should continue to do any more Delta Burke "fat jokes." Some 3,000 people called. Only sixty-five said they wanted Joan to continue doing them. I would like the opportunity to ask those sixty-five people what they think of pulling the wings off of butterflies.

Thursday, January 17, 1991
210 pounds

I've been doing admirably on my diet these last few days. That ugly twelve pounds I'd gained back is soon going to be a thing of the past. Many of my clothes are too big for me again. But you know what's hard to do? It's extremely hard to give away the fat-girl clothes I've "undergrown." Remember how I had inherited boxes and boxes of beautiful clothes? Nice, expensive things? It's like watching a scary movie to think of giving them away. I chew my lips, I breathe deeply, my eyes open wide with horror.

Don't get me wrong; I love to share things. Those clothes meant a new lease on life to *me*. I would be happy to give someone else the "lift" they brought into my life. It's not that, it's—ummmm—*What if I get fat again?* There, I said it. Saving a few boxes of the nicest fat-girl clothes is kind of like the feeling of security you get from putting money in the bank.

But I have been brave. If an article of clothing becomes too big for my delicate, nymphish body, I take a deep breath and give it away. Let someone use those lovely clothes while they are in style. I'm not going to make any grandiose promises of never getting fat again. The struggle is one I must expect to fight every day for the rest of my life. But, somehow, saving a box of fat-girl clothes would seem a bad omen, to say the least.

Saturday, January 26, 1991
206 pounds

I have read my whole diary through three times. I am amazed at the things I have discovered about myself. I am certainly not proud of much of my behavior through the years. It is sheer torture to think of letting the world know what a failure I've been as a wife and mother. I have to believe that someone will be helped by reading these pages, else I could not strip myself naked for all the world to see.

As I read and reread my diary, my soul is hurting for this young woman who was me. I was trying so hard. I continue to struggle daily. I have been keeping this diary for close to nine years. What a hideous and tragic amount of agony I read in these lines. And more pain is hidden between the lines. I hear myself screaming for help, begging for help, dying for help.

I realize at this moment, as I never have before, how much my family has let me down. I'm not angry, but the intensity of my hurt is indescribable. How many times did I plead with Allen? How many times did I tell him exactly what I needed?

Oh, how the world needs re-education. Don't throw up your skinny little arms and say: ''There's nothing I can do to help fat people. When they are ready to lose weight, they will do something about it.'' Oh! What a vicious, insidious lie! All fat people want to lose weight! We ache to be thin. Don't let society fool you one second longer. Big is *not* beautiful. It is ugly and miserable and life-sucking.

I am going to put down in black and white a detailed list of rules my family can follow to help me. I've told them all, countless times, exactly what kind of help I need. But this time, I'm going to post it at strategic points around the house, so they don't forget. I'm sick to death of hearing, ''Oh, you mean I was supposed to . . . ?''

One thing that I came to grips with in this intensive rereading of my diary is this: Obesity is a sickness. I never understood it as thoroughly as I have in the last few weeks. I have tried to divorce myself from me to get a different perspective of my own words and be able to see things in a different light. The obvious intensity of my desire to be thin should have evoked better eating habits. There can be only one reason for failure to do so: Obesity is a sickness. I find myself embarrassed to say that because I don't want anyone to think I'm using "sickness" as a cop-out to eat like a pig. But accepting the fact that I have a sickness is the first step toward recovery. Obesity *is* a sickness. I have a disease. Thank God it is a controllable disease. Only when family members come to accept that reality can they help their loved one.

My friend Kay Johnson is size five-ish. She is an older woman, a living doll. It is hard to believe when I look at her now, but she had a significant weight problem at one time in her life. Like the alcoholic who must remain wary of alcohol, she knows she musn't ever forget food's ability to dominate her. Although Kay has been trim for years, she still prays daily about her eating habits. She recently told me, "I will never forget the feeling of being stuffed. I no longer want to double-cross my body that way. The temptation to overeat is no longer there, because I have learned to get in touch with my body's actual physical hunger—not just some appetizing memory of food. I now pray daily for the desire to eat the right kinds of food."

I, too, will have to be on a "diet," some kind of eating program, for the rest of my life. I have heard countless people say, "I've tried every diet, every professional weight-loss program, every diet pill, every diet drink, fat farms, and diet doctors. I've tried them all, and none of them work." Well, I haven't tried them all. Diet pills are insane, too much of a health risk. Besides, "appetite suppressants" are ludicrous for the fat person. *We are never hungry, so there is never any appetite to suppress!* Fat people nibble all the time. It's a habit. Saying that a foodaholic eats because he is hungry is like saying an alcoholic drinks because he is thirsty! What we foodaholics need is a habit suppressant. I did try that once, in the form of a hypnotist.

I believe that most of an obese person's problem originates

in the mind. That does not mean it is imagined. The problem is indeed real, but I think it could be controlled by fixing something in the brain . . . if scientists could only find that something.

Well, let me tell you, my hypnotist sure couldn't find "that something." What a charlatan. He no more hypnotized me than he helped me lose weight. I mean, I wanted a gold watch swinging before my eyes, right? Ha! No gold watch, no crystal on a ribbon, no lousy button on a piece of yarn, for crying out loud. This quack had thrown up some tacky carpeting on his walls, turned on a cheap tape recorder for background music, and told me to close my eyes while he proceeded to tell me—in a greasy voice—I would get thinner each day.

Big deal. I never became hypnotized. I never even became sleepy. But I wanted it to work. I returned several times. Okay, I was desperate . . . and it *was* about twelve years ago. I am smarter now. Today I would have walked out of that room with a "Who do you think you are kidding here? I mean, where's the snake oil, buster?"

There may be some legitimate hypnotists out there. But it seems to me, if hypnosis really worked, the word would spread so fast, every fat person with a buck in his pocket would be clamoring for an appointment. There would not be one fat person left on the face of the earth.

Tuesday, January 29, 1991
204 pounds

I love reading "Dear Abby" and "Ann Landers." Most of the time, I agree with their answers. They each exhibit plenty of common sense. In both columns I have seen letters dealing with obesity. But because these women are thin, it is impossible for them to answer questions with the psyche of a fat person.

In today's *Oregonian*, Abby showed her "size." The title

above her column read: ACCEPT HER THE WAY SHE IS—FIT AND FAT. *Beeeep!* Incorrect statement. It is impossible to be both fit *and* fat. That is a contradictory and ignorant statement. *Any* doctor will tell you it is unhealthy to be overweight.

The New Medicine Show, by the editors of Consumer Reports books, proclaims that obese women have a greater incidence of cancer of the gallbladder, uterus, ovaries, and breast. Obesity is also associated with colon, rectum, and prostate cancer in men. Gallstones, arthritis, and gout occur much more often in obese people. High blood pressure occurs three times as often, high cholesterol levels occur more than twice as often, and the incidence of diabetes is nearly three times as high. Fit and fat? Preposterous!

For many years, I talked myself into believing I was just fat, not obese. The standard definition of obesity is "20 percent or more overweight." By that definition, if my perfect weight were 130 pounds, I would be obese at 156 pounds. Gee whiz, I'd give my right arm (well, the fat on my right arm) to weigh only 156 pounds. Yet even then, I would be a candidate for all the health problems and diseases I listed above. Yikes!

The contradictory "fit and fat" statement was just the title of the column. The letter writer was also inconsistent. This lady wrote, ". . . I like the way I look and feel. . . . I admit I am about 75 pounds overweight. I've tried all kinds of diets, diet doctors, fat farms, exercise classes—but nothing works for me." Oh please, Abby, reread that paragraph. If this dangerously obese woman, seventy-five pounds overweight, is so happy with the way she looks, why did she try all those different diet programs? Her own words hang her. *Of course* she is unhappy with how she looks! That's why she kept searching for the answer. But there is no quick fix for obesity, so she gave up.

Don't believe anyone who claims to be happy carrying an extra 300 sticks of butter. Why can't skinny people see the tricks we fat people play on ourselves?

The writer said, "Being fat protects me from . . . getting AIDS because men aren't interested in fat women." You didn't comment on that one, Abby, but surely you can feel the frustration in that sentence. For heaven's sake, she wouldn't have mentioned men not being interested in fat women if the lack of interest didn't bother her. People don't write about things they don't think about.

Then, Dear Abby, you quipped the all-time, unthinking skinny-person remark: "I applaud you for accepting yourself as you are." Obesity is a disease, a sickness, Abby. It is physically detrimental, possibly fatal. Yet the *mental* and *emotional* consequences are even more serious, more damaging. Would you applaud the diabetic who refuses to take insulin, or the hearing-impaired man who refuses to wear a hearing aid? Would you applaud the alcoholic who refuses to quit drinking because he "likes himself the way he is"? Then why do you applaud this very sick, obese person who gives up on a cure for her sickness?

If anyone knows the road is hard, I do. But I refuse to give up. I refuse to kid myself into "accepting myself." I have accepted the fact that I have a disease, but I will *not* accept my fat. Fat is unacceptable. Applaud me for my honesty, for wanting to be well someday, for never giving up the goal, even though I falter in my efforts. But please! Don't ever applaud me, or the millions of other sufferers of obesity, for signing our own death warrants.

Finally, Abby, you said, "The National Association to Advance Fat Acceptance . . . is a godsend to people who are tired of being discriminated against because of their size." *Of course* people are discriminated against because of their size! Do you want our next Miss America to weigh 237 pounds? No? But isn't that discrimination?

You are innocently walking along when a man grabs your purse and runs off. A police officer dashes after him. Oops, no, he doesn't dash! He can't dash! He weighs 400 pounds. I want in-shape, physically fit men protecting me and my property. Sure it's discrimination. It's also good sense!

I am fat and I am honest, so I can say this: If I had my choice of hiring two equally qualified persons, I would always choose a thin one over a fat one. I know. I mean, I *know*.

Fat people have a harder time bending over to pick things up off the floor. We avoid it. We have to carefully contemplate exactly how we will move. Fat people walk more slowly. We get out of breath more easily. We cannot think as clearly when we are out of breath. Valuable time is wasted.

Fat people require wider aisles. Some offices are already scrunched up as it is, with little cubicles all over. They cannot accommodate fat people. When a fat person tries to squeeze through a tight place, often either his derriere or his big belly knocks papers off desks and onto the floor. I myself have suffered such embarrassments.

It takes an amazing amount of time to be fat. We are constantly thinking of food, eating food, or preparing food. When a fat person is on the job, that does not mean he can turn off his addiction. The fat person wastes much more time than the thin person—thinking of food, planning for breaks, munching candy bars on the job, and leaving early because he/she is dying to eat. Remember now, I know; I've done it.

If a place of employment supplies uniforms, it costs the employer more to outfit the fat person because larger sizes cost more. Then they wear out faster—between the legs, under the arms, across the stomach—in places where there is constant rubbing.

Upon checking in at an airline, if your luggage weighs over a certain amount, you must pay extra. Why? Because the heavier your luggage, the more fuel it takes to get it to its destination. It works the same way with people. Fat airline stewardesses, on top of all the problems mentioned above, increase their companies' fuel costs, resulting in higher fares. That means higher fares for you and me, kiddo. We're paying the freight for those fat stewardesses' "excess baggage."

I could go on for pages. All I'm saying is, let's be honest. Let's admit that some of the discrimination against fat people is justified. Obviously, a thin person is not *automatically* a better employee than a fat person. (I said "automatically," not "anatomically"! Oh, go ahead and chuckle, it was funny!) But, as I stated, given two *equally* qualified people,

I would *always* hire the thin person. Oops! One exception: I would not hire the thin person to be the fat lady in the circus!

Recently I gathered my family together to formally solicit their support in my weight-loss efforts. I can sense that this time they are earnestly endeavoring to rally around me, and I feel an amazing strength from their help. My biggest surprise is the dedication of four-year-old Tyler. He is always on the lookout for me. He often stays with me in the kitchen, and I am aware that he is being a little policeman on my behalf. Sometimes he even calls me discreetly aside and asks me if what I am eating is on my Daily Menu.

One day, while we were cuddling in bed, I started to tickle him. I laughed, "I'm going to nibble your toes, Tyler." He immediately responded with a cute grin, "No, you can't . . . they're not on your diet!" His great devotion to my cause makes me feel watched after and loved, and that helps me to stick to my diet one more day!

AFTERWORD

Saturday, January 15, 1994
208 pounds

Three years. It was the best three years, it was the worst
three years. No . . . that opener has already been taken!
But the three years since my last entry could be accurately
described as such. I decided it was time to find a publisher
for my diary. I was ready to risk exposing the secrets of my
heart, my weaknesses and failings, and my personal trauma
as an obese person. One of the monumental moments of my
life occurred the day an editor from Warner Books called to
say she was interested in my diary. When I hung up that
phone, I was jumping up and down. I was screaming with
delight. I was running through my house, hugging and kissing
everyone. And I will never forget the day I received my
book contract in the mail with my signature next to *Larry
Kirshbaum's*, president of Warner! What a moment! I mean,
we're talking the chief executive officer of Warner Books!

But other moments during the past three years have not

been so wonderful. I survived the excruciating pain of a herniated disc. I endured the helpless agony of taking care of my father as he daily loses more of his mind to the dreaded Alzheimer's disease. I sobbed my way through the heart-wrenching of having my second child, my first daughter, leave home for Brigham Young University. But my most devastating experience of the past three years concerned my baby brother, Mark. Poor, alcoholic Mark finally took his last drink. On September 25, 1991, I wrote in my diary that Mark had been sober for a year and a half. Tragically, shortly after that entry, Mark again found life too difficult to deal with and once more fell to "that demon rum." Oh Mark! I am so sorry. I know the horrid, out-of-control feeling that overcomes one to the point of suffocation. Then on November 29, 1992, after a few months of continuous drinking, my baby brother was hit by a car while riding his bicycle . . . on his way home from a tavern.

Mark lived for two more months. But he couldn't breathe on his own. He couldn't eat. He couldn't communicate well. He was a quadriplegic. Mark died on January 30, 1993. Through the ordeal of those two long months while Mark was in the hospital, I found several things to be thankful for. I am thankful I could tell him that Warner Books had decided to publish my diary. His eyes brightened for a moment as he looked into mine and mouthed a barely audible "I'm so proud!" I am thankful that after his hideous struggle to live for those two months, my brother Mark was able to leave this life in the condition he had striven so many years to attain—Mark died clean and sober. But most thankful am I that I was able to whisper in his ear, "Mark, I'm going to have another baby. It's a boy. Allen and I want to give him your name. I want you to know that somewhere on this earth is someone who carries your name. It's my gift to you, Mark." His eyes filled with tears, and we cried together for a while.

Steven Mark Green was born April 1, 1993—no foolin'! During that brief period when they lingered at the threshold of heaven together, I like to envision my brother Mark holding

my baby, Steven Mark, and telling him about me. Never was
a baby a more handsome namesake! My dear little Steven
Mark has been the joy of my (Oh! I hate to write this!) old

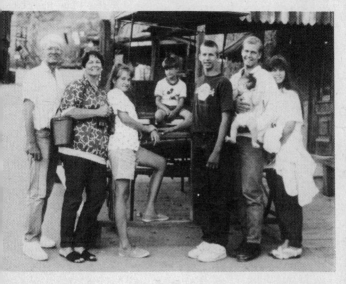

August 1993, 220 pounds. On vacation with my husband and children—I fit on every ride Disneyland had to offer!

age— well, okay, middle age. His birth is yet another strand
in the twine of deep love that binds Allen and me together
. . . through the worst of times as well as the best. In spite
of my mercurial behavior of the past twenty years, Allen has
stuck by me with the tenacity of pitch. My diary is, among
various other things, an amazing love story.

   I also named my precious baby number six after my oldest
brother, Steve. Remember? It was my brother Steve who
challenged me to quit eating chocolate. My brother Steve has
been a great support to me. And I am proud and very thankful
to report that I have met his challenge to stay chocolate

free. Not one M&M, not one chocolate chip, not one bite of chocolate cake, pie, or pudding has passed these lips since September 23, 1991. I believe that forsaking chocolate, in addition to regular spurts of using my Action Plan, has given me the control to keep off the ugly 120 pounds I lost. (I gained about thirty pounds during my pregnancy with Steven Mark, a relatively normal weight gain. And I have lost most of it.)

I look forward with eager anticipation to the new year before me. It is the perfect time to make new commitments. And this new year, I have recommitted myself as never before. True, I have been 100 percent perfect about giving up chocolate. But I still weigh 208 pounds! That is not good . . . or healthy. Don't you think it is about time you gave up a little something else, Rosemary? Yup, I do! So right here, in black and white, I commit to give up any and all candy, pastries, and—want to hear something funny? Even as I am writing these very words, I am thinking of ways to phrase this proclamation so that I can still eat certain goodies. Gee whiz, am I a sicko! Okay, I'll make it all inclusive: no sweets—I mean, *no sweets*, until I weigh less than 150 pounds. If I can give up chocolate for over two years, I can do this thing.

Which brings me to an important thought. We, as a society, have exploded out of control in our sexual promiscuity, in our outrageous mistreatment of children, and in our flagrant practice of substance abuse. In fact, we are out of control in all our physical appetites. Is it really any wonder that we also overindulge in our eating?

We Americans are the fattest country in the world. Surely I am not the only human being who sees the horrible irony of 40,000 babies dying daily from starvation throughout the world . . . while we in America stuff our bodies—sometimes even to the point of immobility. Surely there is something wrong with that picture.

In seriously contemplating my morbid obesity of the past twenty-one years, I have come to some horrible realizations. If I had exercised a little self-control, I could have saved thousands of lives. Recently I decided to donate money to World Relief, an organization dedicated to the alleviation of hunger and poverty worldwide. Every time I forgo some food I crave, *but don't need*, I will contribute the equivalent amount of money to save a baby from starvation. Every time I am tempted by a second dessert, a between-meals taco, or an extra muffin at dinner, I will instead put my pennies in a jar and save some mother from weeping over a tiny, freshly dug grave.

My new slogan is: "Lose a pound . . . Gain a life!" By dieting—a simple act of self-control—I will drastically improve the quality of my life. At the same time, I will be saving lives every day . . . without costing myself one extra penny! It's unbelievable—but true!—that for a meager five cents a day, World Relief can keep a baby alive and healthy. If I will give up just one candy bar, one muffin, or one taco a day, I can keep ten children from starving to death. Sobering thought, isn't it?

So I proposed to World Relief that others might be willing to join me in this plan. They were thrilled. Now I say, let's do it! Let's eradicate excess eating while saving human lives. It will be a double victory! It will be the quintessential win-win situation. We who respond to this challenge will gain a better life, and the world will gain the gift of life.

Join me and mail your tax-deductible diet dollars to the fund established with World Relief for contributions from readers of my book. (Out of every dollar sent to World Relief, an impressive 84.9¢ will actually reach the starving needy!) Send to:

Lose a pound . . . Gain a life!
P. O. Box WRC
Wheaton, IL 60189

To anyone who has now walked the long road of this diary with me, thanks. I hope and pray that at least one of seven things has happened to you as we shared these pages together:

1. You found some comfort from my words, my experiences, my feelings, in that you are not alone. And hopefully, you found a laugh or two.
2. You have the courage to look at the problem/disease honestly, as you stop hiding behind the ''Big Is Beautiful'' myth being promoted by the media . . . and companies with a vested interest in keeping obesity alive and well!
3. You found some motivation to do it. To diet. To gain control of your life. To do something about your obesity: seek counseling, get involved in a support group, try my *Winning at Thinning* Action Plan,^{TM} or devise your own plan—anything to begin the process for a thinner—and better—you. You can do it!
4. You no longer make fun of fat people. Our fat doesn't protect us from others' insensitivity.
5. You gained some insights into the torment of living inside a fat body.
6. You are determined to help your spouse, loved one, or friend conquer this dread disease, this monstrous malady that has overtaken his or her life. You will not give up. You are now aware of how important your help is and what you can do to be part of the solution.
7. You now recognize how easily the poor eating habits of childhood can become the eating disorders of adulthood. You will not use that knowledge as an excuse for gluttony in your adult years, but as an aid to better understand and overcome your weight problem. Furthermore, you will avoid cultivating destructive eating habits in your own children.

Well, I am determined to yet fit into a pair of size-ten jeans. I am determined to yet walk this earth a thin person. I am determined to stand behind my Diary—fat or thin!

May my last words to you be those of glorious hope: I will meet you all again in my sequel to *Diary of a Fat Housewife*, in a book I have dreamed of for years, and already titled: *Thin Again!*

Appendix

Here are some concrete ideas for the dieter and the family or friends of the dieter. I use the pronouns *she* or *her* simply because I am a woman. The pronouns *he* or *him* may always be substituted.

True weight loss requires total commitment. Everyone in the family must come to these realizations:

1. Obesity is a disease. This member of our family has the serious disease of obesity.
2. Nothing is more important than our loved one's getting well, losing weight.
3. In order for our loved one to get well, it will require a new way of life for our whole family. We can help our loved one get used to this new way of life; we can help her "take her medicine."

DO'S AND DON'TS FOR HELPING YOUR SPOUSE, LOVED ONE, OR FRIEND CONQUER HER DISEASE OF OBESITY

NEVER

- Never ask your spouse how much she weighs!
- Never ask your spouse what she just ate or what she is chewing. It is already too late when you see her munching away.
- Never ask when she is going on a diet.
- Never make negative fat comments or jokes about your spouse or about fat people in general.
- Never question money spent on bona fide diet programs.
- Never surprise your spouse with a gift membership to a weight-loss program.
- Never offer an obese person anything to eat. Fat people don't need to be reminded to eat. Sometimes your making the offer is all the fat person needs for an excuse to inhale calories.
- Never ask her to make treats for school, church activities, parties, dinners, or anything else.
- Never push food on an obese person after she has been brave enough to say "No, thanks," just as you wouldn't encourage a recovering alcoholic to "have just one drink"!
- Never belittle "yet another" diet attempt. This one just might work.
- Never yell out in an argument, "Now you have your excuse, why don't you go pig out again?" (Or some such line.)
- Never use any current diet success against the dieter. Example: "Well, if you can be so good on your diet, why can't you clean the house, stop losing your temper [or whatever]?"
- Never tell your obese spouse not to lose too much weight. Someone with a weight problem seldom loses enough weight. Never say she is aiming too low. Never say she would be too thin.
- Never commit to helping your spouse stick to her diet and then fizzle after two days. This obvious lack of caring and support can trigger an astounding eating binge.

- Never deliberately do or say things that you know will trigger an eating response in your spouse. You know what I mean. We all know which "hot buttons" not to push.
- Never leave treats out where your fat spouse can see them. Better yet, never bring home treats for the rest of the family. Sacrifice!
- Never give or send your fat spouse or loved one a box of chocolates, or any fattening food. No exceptions!
- Never take your spouse or loved one to a fast-food restaurant unless you are certain there is an appropriate menu item for her diet.

ALWAYS

- Always be willing to talk with your spouse or friend about her problem, without condemning her. Tell her you love her and want her around for a long time. Read and discuss the medical problems of the obese with her and the advantages of being thin. Ask what you can do to help. Then do what she says!
- Always encourage the children to support her by being on their best behavior, thus alleviating any undue worry or pressure.
- Always encourage your spouse when she says she's going to start a diet, join a support group, get counseling, etc.
- Always encourage her to do her checklist each day before taking time for other things. Nothing is more important than her losing weight.
- Always be ready to work her Daily Checklist with her (or whatever weight-loss plan she chooses). Go over it with her every day, until she has the inner strength to do it on her own. It will take time for her to get well. Weight loss requires total commitment, a new way of life. She needs you to check on her each day to see how she is doing.

- Always be brave enough to apologize after a fight, so she will not have cause to feel justified in eating.
- Always be quick to compliment your spouse anytime you notice her looking better or acting happier. Tell her when you see a waist or feel a curve. Comment when you observe any little thing about her that might make her feel good. She can *never* get too many compliments!
- Always discuss with your fat spouse or loved one exactly what she plans to eat whenever she leaves home. Help her commit ahead of time. Then, whenever possible, stay close by to help her keep her commitment.
- Always remind your spouse or friend when she is coming into her "eating" time of day. Encourage her to be strong and, if she gets crazy to eat something off her diet, to call you instead. If possible, have someone stay with her during that time, making sure she is not alone in the kitchen.
- Always ask her immediately after dinner, "What else are you going to eat tonight?" Encourage her to brush and floss her teeth as soon as she leaves the table.
- Always lock up any sweets or foods that tempt her. Keep careful track of anything that can't be locked up and tell her you know how much is left.
- Always find out the details of her diet. Suggest meals that are good for both of you. If you can't eat the same thing, tell her to fix only her food, that you and the children will take care of your own meals.
- Always remind her to bring her low-calorie seasonings, dressings, and diet pop when going out to eat.
- Always remember, she has a diabolical, lifelong disease. Recovering from any serious disease takes much love, patience, and understanding!

SELF-HELP SUGGESTIONS FOR CONQUERING YOUR DISEASE OF OBESITY

You are dying to be thin. You begin each day with enthusiasm and hope. You try to avoid those fattening foods that you dearly love, but they jump into your mouth, totally without warning. What can you do?

First thing: Start your diet now, this minute. Tomorrow never comes. Don't put it off till next week or after the first of the year. In your committed frame of mind, you can add some important, helpful, stick-to-it principles:

1. If you haven't done so recently, see a doctor and have him recommend a diet. If you're too humiliated to see a doctor at your present weight, use your common sense and eat lots of fresh fruits and vegetables and whole-grain products. Use meat sparingly. Avoid foods high in fat. I'm not a doctor, but I know a person does not need chocolate, maple bars, or ice cream to stay healthy.
2. Set your weight-loss goals realistically. Weigh yourself regularly, and record it. Be honest. No one but you need see the results . . . and you already know how much you weigh.
3. This will be a horrid experience, but take your measurements. I was once about 55–56–57. Not exactly the ideal, hour-glass figure. However, if you're serious about losing weight, it's time to face the fact that you might have to sew two measuring tapes together just to find out how large your hips are!
4. As if taking your measurements didn't make you quite ill enough, now take some pictures of yourself—some honest pictures. In a swimsuit. With no one in front to hide part of you. Holding no baby. Not holding your tummy in till you're blue in the face. Honest pictures. They won't be pretty. Make yourself look at them. Fill yourself with the resolve to never again look that fat.
5. Select a buddy—choose carefully! You need a friend

to whom you can report your progress and problems each day. Your buddy need not be a fat person, but choose someone who can empathize with an addiction. You don't need to tell her your weight, but talk seriously about your problem eating times, your weaknesses. Ask for help and encouragement.

6. Exercise! Check with your doctor before you start any exercise program, to make sure it's right for you. You might want to enlist friends or family to exercise with you.

7. Prepare yourself for some inevitable eating attacks. Have good food available and ready: fresh fruits and vegetables already sliced, skinless chicken already cooked, Sugar Free Jell-O already prepared, any low-calorie food that you like, that you can bite into with a vengeance. Keep sugarless gum on hand for a quick, sweet taste. Make sure your favorite diet soda is chilled. Be prepared.

8. Each day, write down what you plan to eat. Then check off everything you actually consume. Be honest and add anything you ate that wasn't originally listed. Sometimes, just knowing you'll have to add a "forbidden fruit" to your list helps keep it out of your mouth.

9. Ask yourself, before putting anything into your mouth, "Why am I eating this right now?" Get in the habit of being aware of when and why you eat. If you're not genuinely hungry, keep repeating: "The less I eat, the more I lose!" and "This is the fattest day of the rest of my life!"

Saturday, July 15, 1995
135 pounds

I have before me the most important writing assignment of my life. In a few pages I am supposed to tell you how I dropped from 208 pounds (my weight at the end of this diary) down to 135 pounds. A few pages! I want to tell you of the joy, the exultation, *the freedom* I feel as I walk and run in this new, glorious body. I want to describe the spark of excitement that runs through me whenever my husband puts his arm around my waist and whispers in my ear, "I looove your feminine curves!" I want to share the sensuous experience of holding a size-eight silk dress over my head and feeling it slip down over my body . . . and look great on me! I want to somehow portray through words the unequaled thrill of studying my own reflection and proclaiming to myself: "You've done it, Rosemary . . . you reached your goal weight. You got a grip on your horrid, out-of-control, life-ruining, health-destroying eating habits. You conquered the monster within. You will achieve no greater accomplishment . . . or reward . . . in your entire life. I am genuinely proud of you, Woman!"

Yes, that is a tiny fraction of the message I so crave to declare to an overweight-weary nation. But only a tiny fraction . . . because my true feelings about my weight loss are simply magnificent beyond description.

The experience of having my book published has been *mostly* delightful. I have met many wonderful, exciting, and famous people. I have traveled across America—several times—and I have developed a new love and respect for my magnificent country. I have slept in the fanciest hotels and eaten in the finest restaurants this nation has to offer . . . and discovered that I could get used to such luxury reeeeal fast!

So, can you already hear the "BUT . . ." coming? This book experience *has* been delightful . . . but . . . I could never have anticipated the letters. The letters! I have received over a thousand of them. From all over America, from Canada, from Europe, and even from Japan! I have tried to answer each letter personally. Making the time to do that is difficult. But the hardest part of dealing with all these letters is the excruciating pain I feel as I read them. OH! The pain, the misery of obesity! Though I'm thrilled to know my book has meant so much to so many people, I was not prepared for being exposed to the hauntingly familiar pain so many others are still going through.

As I pondered those letters, the nameless masses of obese people became individuals to me. Individuals with their own, unique problems. I have sobbed my way through many letters as I live the pain of my fellow fat friends. Because of my most personal feelings that I disclose in this book, readers of my diary have, in turn, shared with me experiences and emotions they have never disclosed to another human being. Many letter writers even included pictures of themselves, that I might see who I was reading about. And consequently, I have developed a love and feeling of responsibility for these women. It is the screaming pain in those letters that I wish to address here. It is the desperate "How did you do it?" question that I so crave to answer. It is a grave responsibility, and I shoulder it with great apprehension.

My "Moment of Truth" came May 1, 1990. It was on that day that I decided that it was time to publish my diary. And it was the intensive reading and rereading and editing of my diary—in preparation for publication—that finally propelled me into decisive weight-loss action, into taking the steps necessary to empower me to stick to a diet! My friend, you are taking a big step toward weight loss right now . . . as you read this diary.

The cornerstone of my success is simple: There is only one way to lose weight—you must take in fewer calories than you burn in daily activities. That takes into consideration exercise, metabolism, heredity, and fat grams. It is the same formula that has been espoused by doctors for generations. Yup, that means a D-I-E-T . . . diet. Now don't roll your eyes and slam this book shut! Read on for the most illuminating thoughts on dieting that you have ever heard!

While I am a firm believer in diets, I do not believe that every person will be successful with every diet plan. After all, everyone has different food preferences. I strongly advocate making up your own diet menu. Pick out the foods *you* love. One of the diet experts of our day advocates huge portions of oatmeal for beakfast. I HATE oatmeal! It feels slimy and disgusting in my mouth, and I gag every time I take a bite. A diet heavy in oatmeal would never work for me because I would *never* stick to it!

Design your diet to include at least five servings of fruits and/or vegetables daily. Include whole-grain breads and cereals. Don't overlook beans as a wonderful and healthy source of protein. Simply limit your menu to ''X'' number of calories a day. Yup! *Calories do count* . . . so count every one! (Most doctors agree that a diet of 1,000 calories a day will result in a healthy rate of weight loss. But, while you've heard it a million times before, it's still important to remember: Anyone going on a diet should check first with their doctor about what will be safe and effective for them.) What? Count calories . . . not fat grams? Counting only fat grams can get you into dangerous trouble. There are numerous low-fat and fat-free products available today. And they are sometimes more calorie-laden than their higher-fat counterparts. And let's be honest here. For us foodaholics, a ''serving'' is whatever is in front of us. If we open a box of fat-free cookies, within moments we are wearing every calorie in that cute little fat-free box! (And that could easily total some 1400 calories!) And it is *excess calories* that make us fat! And note this **great bonus:** Besides all the other wonderful benefits of reaching your goal weight, you then get to increase the number of calories you eat each day—as you are no longer trying to *lose* weight . . . only to *maintain* it!

So I have come to grips with the fact that I must take in fewer calories. But you know what? Trying to do that can be like living in an eternal hell! Food is everywhere. Like air. You cannot open a magazine, turn on the TV, ride down the street, or listen to the radio without experiencing umpteen tantalizing food advertisements. Almost any function you attend offers tempting goodies.

Food is a horrible addiction from which to break free. I suffered twenty long years of morbid obesity. I thought of suicide numerous times. I hated going anywhere. I struck out at my children . . . both verbally and physically. (Oh! How my heart aches as I write this!) My marital relationship suffered . . . both emotionally and physically. Now, as I read my diary, I am amazed that I survived. But somehow, the spark of the Divine that is within each of us stayed lit within me. It inspired me to try over and over to conquer the addiction. A modest estimate is that I started dieting over 20,000 times. That's *twenty thousand* times! I thank God daily that I started the twenty thousand and first time! I say to you, my fat friends—never stop starting. Never, never, NEVER STOP STARTING!

Besides counting calories, there were three key principles critical to my weight-loss success:

1. HONESTLY ADMIT THAT OBESITY IS AN UNDESIRABLE CONDITION! No problem can be solved until it is faced. Obesity is, without question, a serious health problem. If for no other reason that that, I must eradicate it from my life. And come on, this is America, the land of the free and the brave . . . and the money hungry. If obesity were really a happy, sought-after condition, there would be plenty of businesses advertising: ''For only thirty dollars a month

we guarantee to add yet another chin to your neck, double your fat rolls, and increase your thighs by ten inches!" Doesn't that just sound bizarre? Think about it!

2. ACCEPT TOTAL RESPONSIBILITY FOR THE SHAPE OF YOUR BODY! I had to come to grips with the fact that there is no calorie count in an argument with my husband. No calorie count in a misbehaved offspring. No calorie count in an unhappy childhood memory. Only excess calories make me fat. And only *I* bend my elbow to stuff in those excess calories! When pressures and stress propel me—like a race car driver at top speed—directly toward the fridge, it is *I, Rosemary*, who must mentally, even audibly, scream out, "NOOOOOO! I will not eat to calm myself. It has never yet solved one lousy problem for me. I am only using this frustrating experience as an excuse to do something that feels good for a nanosecond. If eating felt like getting my fingers slammed in the door—I would never have gotten fat in the first place. Neither would anyone else. I refuse to wallow in the abuse of the excuse one second longer!"

3. PRACTICE ENVIRONMENTAL CONTROL! Please, please, please, my dear, fat friends: Pay particular attention to this principle. It has worked miracles in my life. It was only after reaching my goal weight of 135 pounds that I came to understand the critical importance of environmental control. I call it practicing "the common sense of self-defense," and it has not only enabled me to lose the weight—but to keep it off.

Finally, I realized that the typical "Here's a diet . . . now stick to it" line from the doctors simply wasn't enough. I faced the fact that willpower, applied at the wrong point, had failed me for years. Willpower alone simply *isn't* enough. At least not in the conventional sense. I still cannot trust myself alone with a cheesecake. I am afraid I would eat the whole thing. So should I throw up my arms and give up? Or should I practice "the common sense of self-defense"— a conscious effort at environmental control where food is concerned—and NEVER ALLOW MYSELF TO BE ALONE WITH A CHEESECAKE!? You see, I have discovered that we fatties must look further than traditional *will-power* for a solution. We must implement a little ol' *brainpower*! We must determine which link is our weak link in the stimulus-response chain that leads to overeating. At which point in the chain can we expect our willpower to fail?

After twenty years I faced the fact that I simply can't control myself once the maple bar is in my hand. At that point, it is not my fault if I eat it. It is literally beyond my control. Like the alcoholic sitting at a bar with his favorite drink in front of him, once that stupid maple bar is in my hand, I am a goner. BUT . . . I *did* have control before I bought the greasy sucker. Or before I walked into the store. Or before I got out of my car. Or before I stepped into my car. Heck, I knew I was going to buy that life-wrecking hunk of sugar and grease before I sneaked out of my house. *That is where willpower must be applied!* When the first wicked thought of excess calories enters the brain—that is the place to nip it! Benjamin Franklin said, "It is easier to suppress the first desire than to satisfy all that follow it." And Mark Twain said, "It is easier to stay out than to get out." So, I have made a commitment to me: I am Rosemary. I am a foodaholic. I must never again go into a grocery store alone. Allen now does all the grocery shopping. Why incite my millions of food-addicted taste buds unnecessarily . . . while I am alone and vulnerable in the store, with a whole cartful of food? In which a package of cookies, a half gallon of ice cream, or a dozen candy bars could easily hide . . . till the trip home? If I follow that rule, I will never again buy a stupid maple bar. "The common sense of self-defense." The sweet sound of thin and healthy for life! You see, I have become like the alcoholic who was smart enough to get out of the tavern!

Think of the extremes to which a basketball coach goes to win a game. He makes his team carefully scrutinize a video-tape of their latest game. They study each move. They discuss each player's strengths and weaknesses. They plan strategies and plays to improve their next game. Their next *game*. All this planning and scheming . . . for a *GAME*!

It finally dawned on me that I must show at least as much respect for my health, my happiness, my life . . . as a coach does for a lousy basketball game. It was at that moment when "thinness" and a healthy body became a possibility for me! I now analyze every "food mistake" that I make: Every time I eat out of control, I analyze "why" I indulged . . . and try to never repeat that self-destructive behavior.

I started practicing self-defense by cleaning out my environment. I attacked my kitchen like the enemy it is! I discarded any overly tempting, patently unhealthy foods: potato chips, candy, pastries, most crackers, ice cream, and nuts.

WAIT! I already know what you're thinking (I played the fat game for twenty-two long years): "But I can't throw away money like that, and besides, my children need treats." To which I reply, "Phooey!" This will be the best-spent money you have ever known! It will be an investment in you and your new way of life. If the tempting garbage food is in your home—you will eat it. It is that simple. My friend and personal tutor, Dr. Jerry Darm, calls it "The Arm's Length Rule: If it is within arm's length . . . you will eat it." You are not a bad person to eat it, but you are a stupid person to have it in your home. Really now, who *needs* potato chips? Who is healthier for eating potato chips? Do you honestly want your sweet babies to put those grease-laden, unhealthy morsels into their beautiful little bodies? Do you actually want their precious little arteries becoming clogged with life-taking plaque? I again quote Dr. Darm: "We need to think of a French fry . . . as a cigarette!"

To which I add this killer thought—think of what we do at Christmas, Valentine's Day, and Easter: "Here, my darling child, with your beautiful, healthy little body, here's a special chocolate treat. It's made from 50% grease and 50% sugar . . . I love you!" That doesn't sound like love to me! What chance do those children have at staying trim and healthy? Why do we do what we do when we know what we know? I mean, any decent parent would be appalled at the prospect of offering their child a cigarette or a drink of beer. Why? Because it is unhealthy for them! But it's somehow okay, perfectly acceptable, to offer them globs of fat. So, cleaning out your environment will benefit *anyone who lives under your roof*!

But beware! Do not throw those garbage foods into the garbage can . . . we both know they are too easily retrievable. Okay, here's one of my favorite lines—think it over carefully: Grind them or flush them . . . or you're going to wear them.

I had much more control over my food intake the instant I gutted out my kitchen. But now, with a sirens' song, the soft, fresh, low-fat, good-for-me bagels called out to me. And the nutritious, vitamin-fortified cold cereal. And the wholesome bread. I would clench my fists and grit my teeth whenever I passed the cupboard they were in. I can eat a whole package of bagels in one sitting . . . or a whole box of cold cereal. Then one day, when I heard those bagels singing, "Come, Rosemary . . . come, My Pretty, and indulge in my delectable softness and flavor . . ." I came. I came with screwdriver and hasp. Yes! I installed a lock on that stupid cupboard. I couldn't take the fight any longer. Why should I? Instead of facing the daily challenge of not eating too much of even the "healthy foods," I practiced the common sense of self-defense by installing a lock! (Hey, a calorie is a calorie, and 3500 excess "healthy" calories will put a pound on me just as quickly as the unhealthy ones will!) A simple combination lock solved the problem. Everyone in the family knows the combination—EXCEPT ME—and is completely supportive of my efforts to stay trim and healthy.

Sadly, environmental control is not so easy outside my home. But I must never forget that I once weighed 320 pounds! So I created a custom, hands-on, diet-motivation plan for myself—my *Winning at Thinning!*™ Action Plan. In it I documented my successes and failures. I kept track of the things I did that helped me fight this addiction, and made a valiant effort to make them a part of my daily routine. (Still do.)

Every day, Allen and I spend about half an hour working my *Winning at Thinning!*™ Action Plan. It offers amazing "sticking" power! One of my favorite parts is "thinking thin.'' When I was fat, I would close my eyes and dream of thinness. Or I would pore over pictures of thin, beautifully dressed women and imagine myself looking as chic! *Now* I "think thin" (or should I say *"live thin"*?) while I shop for those beautiful clothes . . . *and they fit me!*

Another critical item in my Action Plan is the listing of what I will eat for the day. I think ahead. I check my calendar for any wedding or baby showers, parties, business luncheons, church socials. I *know* there will be food at such events. So I must be prepared. I must practice self-defense. Since Allen is usually with me, he is a great help. I tell him, before we step into *the lion's* mouth, just exactly how many calories I can put into *my* mouth. If I screw up and overeat (who . . . ME?) then I calorie-balance the next day. In other words, I eat fewer calories to make up for excess eaten the day before. The body is a wonderfully forgiving machine that allows us to do this.

A third key element in my Action Plan keeps me looking my best, no matter my weight. I keep my hair washed and curled, my legs shaved, my nails polished. I discovered that looking good is a critical component of feeling good and is a significant boost to that important word *willpower*!

My Action Plan evolved over the many years that I wrote my Diary. It can be a significant, motivational boost to any diet. When I first met Dr. Darm, I had lost a total of 140 pounds on my own, 25 in the two months just before I met him. He suggested that I enroll in a doctor-supervised liquid diet program. I had never been part of any formal weight-loss program before. I had never even really considered it. Dr. Darm pointed out that doing so would give me a much broader perspective of the whole weight-loss experience. As I debated whether to try it, he made me an offer I couldn't refuse: He offered to pay for my participation in the program. Amazing how easily that did the trick! As part of the program, I had to attend weekly group meetings to help inform and motivate me. Bottom line: It was a great way to diet. It was probably the easiest weight-loss experience of my life. I lost my last 45 pounds on that program, achieving my goal weight of 135 pounds on December 27, 1994. But it wasn't a magic cure—I worked darn hard. I continued using my Action Plan regularly. I sacrified Halloween sweets, my traditional Thanksgiving feast, and Christmas goodies! (Looking back, I realize that it was a smart time to diet!) Now, I have heard all the stories about how you can supposedly never keep off weight lost on a liquid diet. But I am intelligent enough to know that I will not gain back that 45 pounds simply because I lost it in that reputedly unorthodox manner. Any claim to the contrary is clearly an excuse for the ex-dieter to return to her gluttonous ways. If I ever regain *one pound*, it will be because I started eating too darn much again.

Well, I could go on for pages about all the things I have done to maintain this weight loss. For pages! And that is exactly what I am doing in working on my next book, *Thin Again!* For me, it is crucial to never forget how it felt to be so fat . . . and how great it feels to be thin! I must never go back to that depressing and limiting lifestyle. The miserable memories of that time help motivate me to keep going, to keep counting calories, to keep writing diary entries.

I feel compelled to share with you my most disappointing moment in the production and promotion of this book. It occurred when Hugh Downs made the following comment in his introductory remarks to a rerun of a segment featuring me on ABC's *20/20*. Without having talked to me for so much as a second, he bluntly proclaimed: "She is a former obese person who has no mercy for people who say they just can't lose weight." Oh! how my heart ached at his callous, unfair remark. I couldn't help recalling the hundreds of letters I had answered from women all over the world. The aching in my hands and shoulders as I bent over my desk, pen in hand, to try and offer some advice and consolation. The hot tears I shed as I read of their suffering, or talked with them on the phone. The many late hours when my eyes were heavy and my head bobbed. The countless times I had to tell baby Steven, "Not now, Honey, Mommy is busy answering letters." The lying awake nights worrying about these new friends who were looking to me for help. The feeling of love and responsibility for them—as if they were my own children. The hundreds of dollars in postage and long distance phone calls that added up as I agonized with these women. Yes, after spending all that emotion, time, and money—it hurt bigtime to be accused of having no mercy!

If there is anyone else out there who has come to a false conclusion about how I feel toward obese people—now that I have reached my goal weight—please know this: I suffer this dread disease right along with them. I still have my out-of-control days. I still have to count my calories. I still struggle not to pull in when I pass a fast-food restaurant. And most important, I still feel a real, physical pain for any sufferer of this horrible disease of obesity. I desire to help in any way that I can. Remember: *Winning at thinning* is not a destination . . . it is a lifelong journey. Read my Diary and join me along the steep climb! I am convinced that helping each other is the only way to ultimate, sustained success.

P.S. I am still chocolate-free! It's been almost four years. It *can* be done!

By the year 2000, 2 out of 3 Americans could be illiterate.

It's true.

Today, 75 million adults… about one American in three, can't read adequately. And by the year 2000, U.S. News & World Report envisions an America with a literacy rate of only 30%.

Before that America comes to be, you can stop it… by joining the fight against illiteracy today.

Call the Coalition for Literacy at toll-free **1-800-228-8813** and volunteer.

Volunteer Against Illiteracy. The only degree you need is a degree of caring.

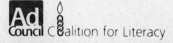

Ad Council   Coalition for Literacy